# HERBS

## THE HEALING NATURE

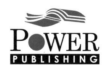

P☉WER
PUBLISHING

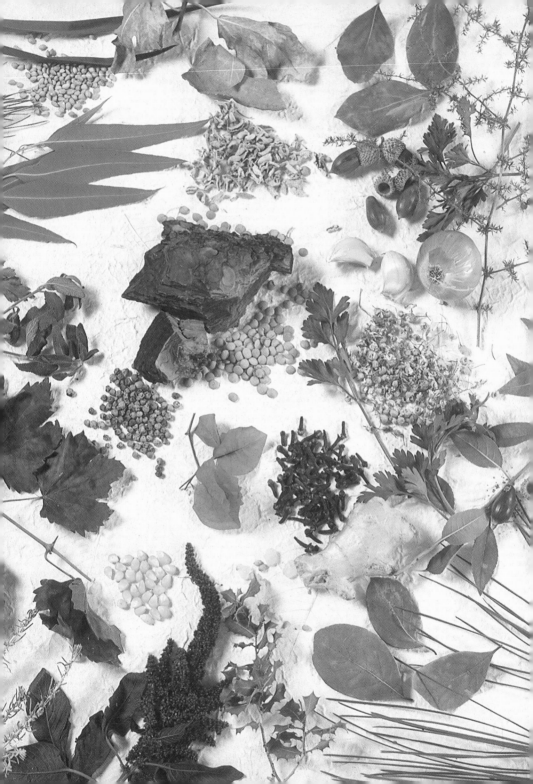

this plant keep in life a few millions of patients with heart problems.

Herbal medicine has its roots in three major systems: the traditional Chinese medicine which is actually part of the Far Eastern medicine, Ayurveda and Western Herbal medicine that basically started in ancient Greece and Rome and eventually expanded to the rest of Europe.

Chinese medicine, as well as Ayurveda, have developed into complicated diagnostic and healing systems through the centuries. Western herbal medicine consists of a collection of traditional recipes and treatments.

During the last few years, the interest of herbs and their healing properties has shown a remarkable increase in the Western world, where huge pharmaceutical companies produce and supply the market a wide variety of chemical medicines.

For example, St John's Wort is now being widely used for the treatment of mild to moderate cases of depression, replacing Prozac, the most widely used antidepressant. Clinical studies have indicated that St John's Wort is at least as effective as Prozac in cases of mild to moderate depression. The major difference between the two is that St John's Wort does not have any side effects, it is not addictive and in general it is more safe.

There are of course a lot of other examples like this, such as herbs helping people with high cholesterol levels, diabetes, heart conditions, etc. On the other hand, there is a growing number of herbs that are used as supplements such as Ginseng, Garlic and many others.

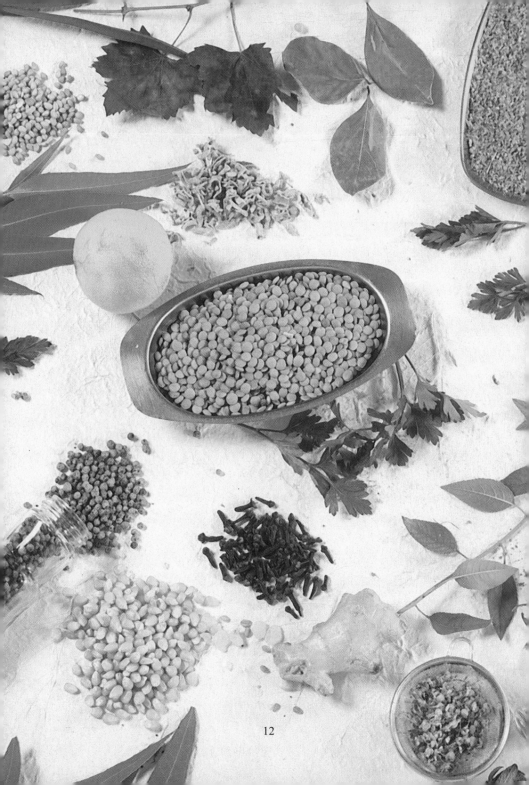

12

use honey instead of sugar.

## DECOCTION

Decoctions are prepared in a similar way to teas and we use them to extract the active ingredients from roots, seeds and the bark. Because these parts of the plant are hard, we simmer them in the water while boiling until the active ingredients of the herb are released in the water. The boiling time ranges but we can say in general that we leave them to boil until the volume of the water is reduced to half its original volume. It is better to cover the water when left to cool down, so that the volatile ingredients of the decoction do not escape with the fumes.

## HERBAL OILS

Herbal oils are used externally for massages. They are prepared using fresh herbs which contain volatile (easily evaporated) oils. Crush the fresh herbs with a mortar and pestle. Add some olive oil (1 liter of olive oil to 100 grams of the herb) and leave the mixture in a warm place, away from sunlight for three days. Drain the herbs and store the oil, which has been enriched with the volatile oil of the herb in dark, air tight, glass containers for future use.

A second category of herbal oils, the volatile oils are used both externally as well as internally, always diluted in water and always after professional advice. These oils are extracted with the method of distillation and are highly concentrated.

## TINCTURES

Tinctures are highly concentrated liquid extracts of the herbs. They are quite easy to prepare and one of the best ways to store the ingredients of a herb for future use. They are prepared mixing the powder of very finely ground leaves or flowers in alcohol. Alcohols used are usually vodka, brandy or pure alcohol. Use enough alcohol to cover the herbs completely and keep the closed container in a warm place, away from direct sunshine. Allow the herbs to stand in alcohol for two weeks, shake it daily and add alcohol whenever it does not cover the herbs. Drain the herbs from the alcohol, pressing the herbs to release any liquid they have absorbed and store it in a dark, glass container.

Tinctures are usually diluted in some water. In this way the alcohol is diluted and the patient does not feel it. It is accustomed to start the tincture on a new moon and drain the herbs on the next full moon so that the moon helps in the extraction of the curative ingredients of the herbs.

## SYRUPS

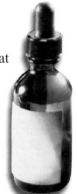

Syrups are usually used for treating cough and throat diseases but it is also a very convenient way to give a herb to small children. Put 100 grams of the herb in one liter of water and simmer until the volume of the water is reduced to half its original volume. Drain the herbs and add 100 grams of honey stirring it for a while until it becomes a uniform thick liquid. We can add a few drops of lemon or orange juice to add flavor to the syrup.

## SALVES / OINTMENTS

Salves and ointments are always used externally for the treatment of skin diseases but also for other diseases such as arthritis, rheumatism and even colds. For example, Vick vapor rub is used for easing breathing in flu. They are also used as cosmetics and deodorants. Boil a handful of the herb in 3 to 4 cups of water for 15 minutes for leaves or flowers or 30 minutes for roots. Drain the herbs and add 150 grams of olive oil in the water and continue simmering until all the water vaporizes. Then boil 50 grams of beeswax and simmer it until it reaches the same temperature as the oil. Mix the oil with the beeswax and continue simmering until you have a uniform cream. Pour the cream in glass containers and leave it to cool entirely.

## CAPSULES

Some herbs are very efficient but their taste is not so tasteful so capsules are used to cover the taste of the herb. They are also the best way to take herbs for a long period of time or for those that don't have the time to prepare their herbs. Crush the herbs into powder or very fine pieces and fill the capsules. You can get your empty capsules from the market. We usually use small capsules size "0" or medium size "00".

## POULTICE

Grind the herbs, moisten them with a few drops of water and apply it directly to the affected area. Sometimes you can use the fresh, crushed leaves in a cloth or even use the decoction of the herb to wet the cloth and apply the cloth to the affected area.

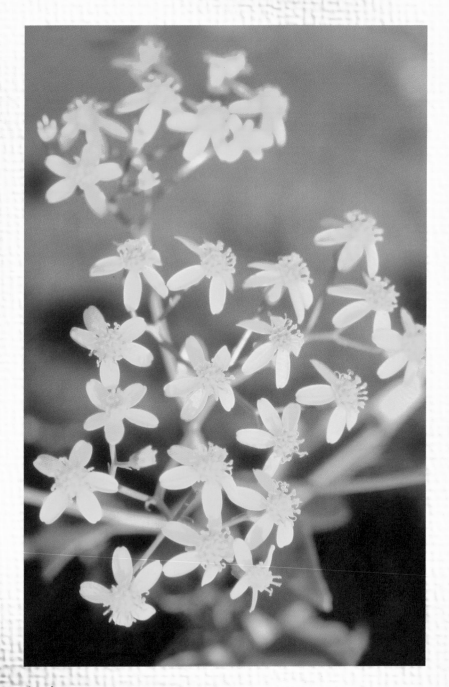

**Agrimony**

# Agrimony
*Astringent, tonic, diuretic,*

**Scientific Name:**
Agrimonia eupatoria of the Rosaceae family

**Parts Used:** the whole plant, especially the leaves and its yellowish flowers.

**USES:** Agrimony is used as a treatment for:
- Diarrhea
- Diabetes
- Kidneys
- Sore Throat
- Pharyngitis
- Inflammation

External use - it is used locally against the bites of bees, insects and snakes as well as for removing thorns from our skin. It is also used in lotion form at wounds and ulcers and in gargle solution to strengthen the pituitary glands of the mouth and the throat. It is also used in bruises, skin rashes, swellings and against fractures.

Internal use - used to promote digestion to reduce stomachaches, for arthritis or rheumatism, for cough, tonsillitis and even common cold. It is considered to be very helpful for the cure of winter colds and high fever. Since it is diuretic, it will help people with gall bladder stones. It is anti-diabetic, anti-emetic and muscle strengthener.

## PREPARATION & DOSAGE

The dried herb is ground into grain and is boiled to produce extract.

Infusion - Put one teaspoon of dried agrimony root, leaves or flowers in one cup of boiled water and leave it for about 15 minutes. Strain the water and add some honey or glycerine for taste. This infusion is a good blood cleanser and you can have up to one cup daily. Alternatively, we can put one or two teaspoons of Agrimony flowers in one liter of hot water for 15 minutes. We drink it in cases of cystitis, kidney or liver problems and gastroenteritis without sweetening it.

Poultice - we make hot poultices with its leaves, which are very soothing in cases of migraines, neuritis and fractures.

We can take Agrimony orally for diarrhea or inflammations of the mouth or throat. The typical daily dosage is about three grams (one and a half teaspoons) of the herb or equal dosage of pharmaceutical preparations.

## OTHER USES

We can leave the root of agrimony is some water for half an hour and then drink the water. This drink is very helpful in cases of constipation and will also strengthen the liver. If we put some leaves of Agrimony in our bath, they will help our muscles to relax.

## SIDE EFFECTS

Agrimony contains tannin, so the use of greater than the recommended dosage may lead to constipation and other digestive problems.

## HISTORY

Agrimony was widely known throughout the history of medicine. There is evidence that it was used from ancient times from almost all civilizations. It was actually often considered a cure all herb.

The ancient Greeks were using it to cure the eye diseases. Preparations of Agrimony were used to cure diarrhea, malfunctions of the gall bladder, the liver and the kidneys. It was also used externally for wound healing, while in England it was used on snake bites and skin rashes. In North America the Indians used it against high fever with great success.

22

# Almond

*Emollient, diuretic, anti-diabetic,*
*tranquilizer, antipyretic.*

**Scientific Name:** Prunus amygdalus of the Rosaceae family.

**Parts Used:** Leaves, flowers, fruits and their skin.

USES: There are two main categories of almonds: sweet almonds and bitter almonds. All preparations using bitter almonds are intended for external use only and are not to be taken orally.

The tea of sweet almonds is used against whooping cough, liver insufficiency and prostate hypertrophy. As an emollient it is prescribed for first-degree burns.

Diuretic - the decoction of its leaves is a good purgative.

Antidiabetic - it helps lowering the sugar levels of diabetics.

Antipyretic - it is sedative in fevers, inflammations of the uric system and skin irritations. It is also used as a tranquilizer in nervous breakdown.

## PREPARATION & DOSAGE

Tea - put two teaspoons flowers or fresh leaves of Almond in a cup of hot water and leave it for 15 minutes. Drain it and drink it hot.

Decoction - Boil two handfuls of Almond fruit skin in one litre of water for 20 minutes and filter the water. Drink it in small cups for as long as the cough holds. It is very effective in cases of cocitis or whooping cough.

## OTHER USES

Bitter almonds contain prossic acid which is a strong poison therefore be careful not to take any bitter Almonds preparation orally. Nevertheless, baths with bitter almond porridge are very sedative to pain

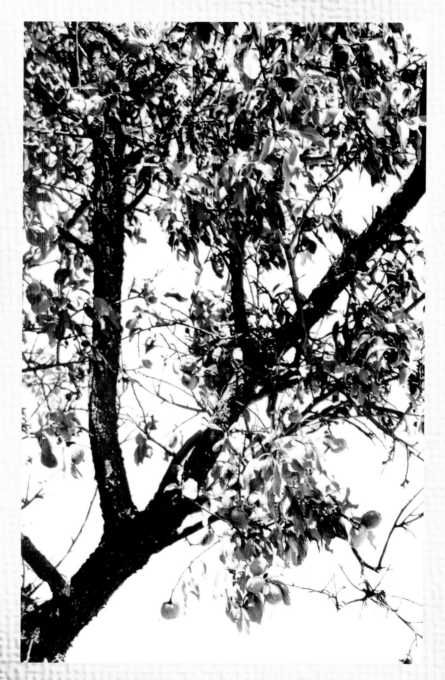

**Almond** 24

especially migraines, colic of the kidneys and the liver, reumatic pain and stomach sourness. For people with sensitive skin there are bitter Almond soaps available in the market.

## SIDE EFFECTS

Bitter Almonds are dangerous and may even cause death if we eat 50-60 of them at the time. Still, not all people react the same to their poison so it is better not even to taste a bitter Almond.

Sweet Almonds may also cause some troubles if we eat a lot like indigestion, sleeplessness and even skin rashes. An antidote to Almond is plain sugar but in serious cases of poisoning we must definitely cause vomit and may be use Atropine.

## HISTORY

Almond tree was originally grown in Central Asia and evidence shows that it has been cultivated in China and Persia for more than 35 countries. Today it is found in a lot of places around the world but there are some parts of the planet that will never grow almond trees since it requires the strong sun of the equatorial areas of the planet. The flowering almond tree offers a wonderful view and has been worshiped by poets and painted by famous painters. It was also one of the most favorite subjects of the ancient Chinese silkscreen printers. Evidence of its medical use was found in Hippocratic notes who used Almond's leaves and fruit in a lot of treatments.

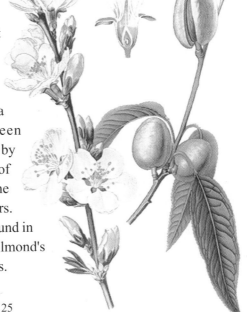

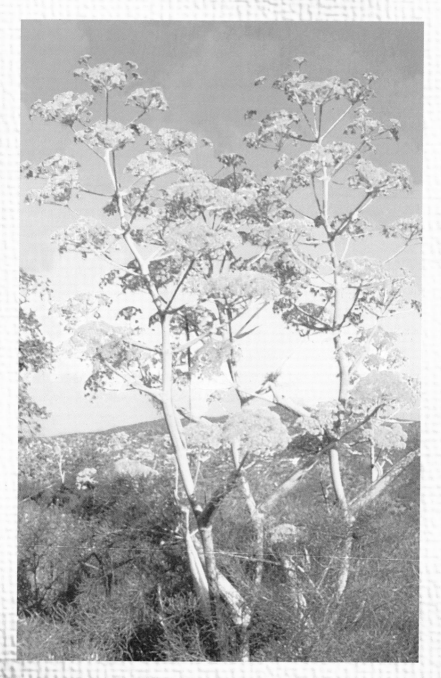

**Angelica**

# Angelica

*Tonic, Sedative, Fights anorexia.*

**Scientific Name:** Angelica archangelica of the Umbelliferae family.

**Parts Used:** Seeds, leaves and roots.

**USES:** Angelica is used as a treatment for:

- Menstrual pains
- Anemia
- Fatigue
- Anorexia
- Thrombosis
- Psoriasis and arthritis
- Gland swelling

Angelica is often described as the "Female Ginseng" due to its many curative properties on women. It is probably the best herb used for the menstrual period, it soothes the pain and eliminates the spasms of the bosom. Angelica also helps women during the menopause period.

The upper part of the root helps in blood reproduction and that is why it is used as a tonic and as a treatment of anemia. The ends of the root are used in cases of thrombosis of the arteries in emergency situations, after an accident.

## PREPARATION & DOSAGE

Tea - (for all the uses mentioned above) heat one teaspoon of dried root or seeds of Angelica and leave it to boil for 1-2 minutes. Drain the tea and cover it with a cloth for 15 minutes.

A more convenient way to take the herb is in powder form that has been previously enclosed into capsules. The normal dosage is two capsules per day (3-4 grams) but in more serious cases you can take up to 3 capsules daily.

## OTHER USES

The root of Angelica is often used to add flavor to certain alcoholic drinks especially gins and liqueurs. Because of its distinctive flavor, Angelica is also widely used in confectioneries and during the past few years Angelica is being cultivated industrially.

## HISTORY

There is an ancient legend that says that Angelica has been revealed by Archangel Michael to humanity to save the world from a terrible epidemic. And in reality, it is considered by lot of people as the king of herbs. The Chinese have been using Angelica for thousands of years now, mainly to soothe and cure female problems. Still, its use in not limited to women since it has been also used for men with heart diseases, hypertension and circulatory problems. Parkinson revealed in 1629 that he was convinced that Angelica was the best of all medical plants.

During the early years of Christianity, the herb was greatly respected and was considered a gift from God that was given to cure all evil diseases. In some places of the world it is still known as the "root of the Holy Spirit".

# Anise

*Digestive, stomachic, stimulant, carminative.*

**Scientific Name:** Pimpinella anisum of the Umbelliferae Family.

**Parts Used:** Seeds and its essential oil.

**USES:** Anise is used for the treatment of:
- Indigestion
- Flatulence
- Intestinal colic
- Asthma
- Cough
- Stomach Pain
- Toothache

External Use - the volatile oil of Anise can be used against scabbies and lice.

Internal Use - Anise is widely used to relieve from cough especially hard, dry cough. It is also used for the treatment of bronchitis and asthma, and its stomachic properties have been recognized from ancient times, when it was used to relieve from stomach pains, flatulence, intestine colic and indigestion. Anise is still being used today for the above disorders.

Stimulant - Anise has been found to stimulate the function of the heart, the lungs, the liver and even the brain.

Children - Anise tea is very effective against children intestine colic and also infantile catarrh or cold.

Woman - Its seeds are galactogogue and will increase the production of milk in nursing women while, on the other hand, it is sometimes used to relieve women from menopausal discomforts.

Men - Anise has been lately being used for the treatment of some forms of prostate cancer.

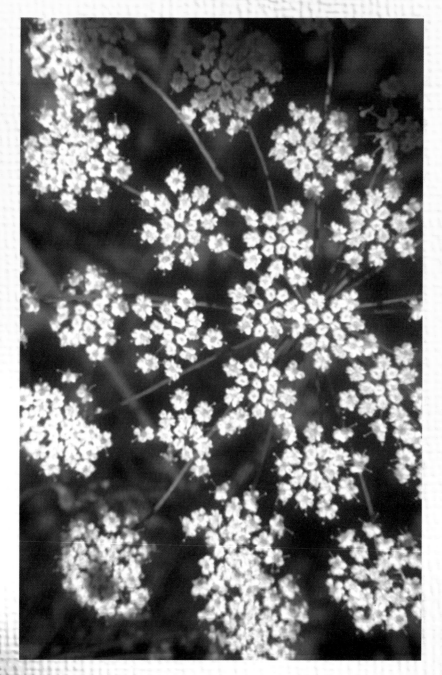

**Anise**

## OTHER USES

In cases of toothache, drop a few drops of the essential oil of Anise in a cup of water and gargle the tooth in pain with it.

Anise is widely used in the production of aromatic drinks like the well known Greek ouzo and also to add flavour in medicines.

## PREPARATION AND DOSAGE

Infusion - In cases of insomnia drink a cup of milk where you have droped a few seeds of Anise, just before you go to bed.

Decoction - boil one teaspoon of Anise seeds in a cup of waters for about 10 minutes, drain it and drink it hot twice daily. It is very effective against stomach pain and intestine colic. For intestine colic in children, you can boil the seeds in milk instead of water and again give it to the child twice daily.

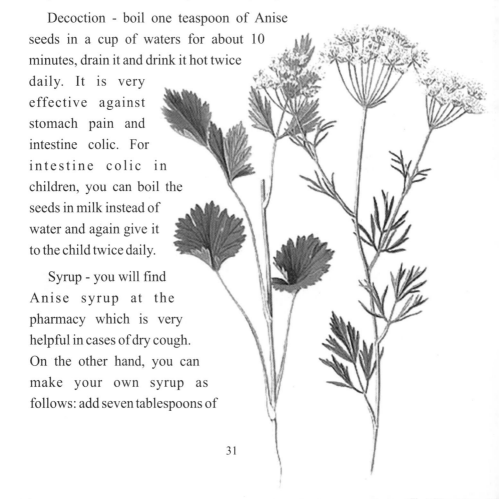

Syrup - you will find Anise syrup at the pharmacy which is very helpful in cases of dry cough. On the other hand, you can make your own syrup as follows: add seven tablespoons of

Anise seeds to one litre of water and boil it until it evaporates to half its initial quantity. Drain the seeds and add four tablespoons of honey and another four tablespoons of glycerine (as a preservative).

Your syrup is considered to be memory strengthening. To improve your memory, you can also drink two tablespoons of the decoction three times daily.

In cases of flatulence you have to drink the decoction in small sips just before each meal.

## SIDE EFFECTS

It is not recommended to be used during pregnancy and also if your doctor has prohibited the use of birth control pills, avoid taking Anise because it has some estrogen activity. Estrogen is suspected to be the cause of migraine headaches, abnormal blood clotting and even promote the development of certain types of brain tumors. Large quantities of Anise oil (that is, several tablespoons at once) may cause nausea and vomiting.

## HISTORY

Anise is a herb known to be used by people for a lot of centuries now. Ancient Greek physicians, including Hippocrates, were using it for common cold and the flu. In ancient Rome, Anise was used in the production of Anise cake that was eaten after their big feasts as an aid for digestion. Historically, Anise attracted people because of its pleasant flavor and it was used all over Europe for indigestion, flatulence, colic and nausea. The herb was also known in ancient China where it was used against indigestion and flatulence as well as a breath freshner.

# Apple
*Digestive, antioxidant, laxative, dentifrice*

**Scientific Name:** Pyrus malus of the Pomaceae family.

**Parts Used:** leaves, buds, flowers, bark and fruit.

USES: Apple is used for the treatment of:
- Constipation
- Sore eyes
- Fever
- Rheumatism
- Kidneys
- Pharyngitis
- Indigestion
- Anti-toxication

"An Apple a day, keeps the doctor away", an old saying that probably contains a lot of truth. Apples are rich in malic and tartaric acid, vitamin C and a variety of salts like salt of potash, soda, lime, magnesium, iron etc. These ingredients help the body get rid of the toxicities stored in it and at the same time improve the function of the liver and neutralize the acids produced by digestion. This is also why Apple and Apple juice help people trying to lose weight.

The acids contained in the fresh fruit not only help in the digestion of the apple itself but promote the digestion of other food as well, if we eat them half an hour before each meal. And although about 80% to 85% of the Apple is water, the sugar it contains is quickly metabolised providing energy and warmth to the body.

Apple juice, without any sugar, reduces the stomach acidity and corrects sour fermentation due to the fact that it is quickly transformed into alkaline carbonates. Apple juice is also an excellent diuretic with beneficial properties to the kidneys. In fact, a population study in Normandy, where the no-sugared Apple juice is a favourite drink,

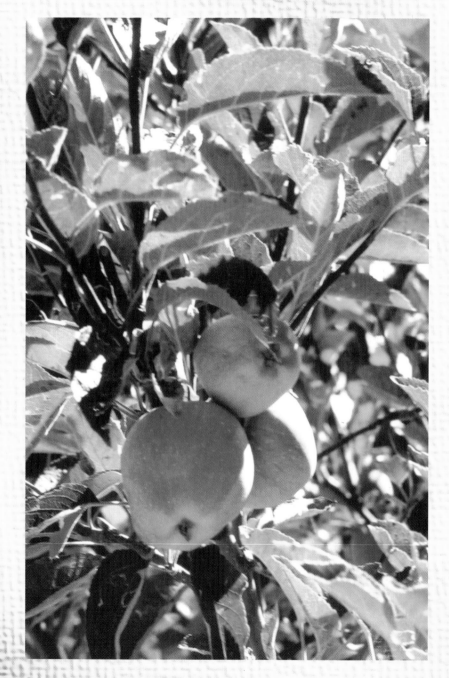

**Apple**

showed that not a single case of kidney stones has been mentioned in that area for the last forty years.

Apple is also beneficial to our teeth. Apples not only clean the teeth with their acids but also push the gums back in a way that the borders get cleaned from food deposits.

Sour, ripe Apples are used against constipation. Eating them before going to bed will act as a laxative and at the same time it will calm down the stomach promoting a good night's sleep.

Scientific research has proved that glucoside, a substance extracted from the bark and the root of Apple tree and other trees of the same family, has the property to induce diabetes. In fact these results were derived from animal experiments but researchers are confident that the same substance will have similar effects to human diabetics.

The bark of the Apple tree is also used against fevers and sometimes as a tonic.

The leaves, buds and flowers are excellent diuretics.

## OTHER USES

Sour Apples will produce cider, which is very useful to the peptic system. Of course ripe Apples have been used in the production of delicious apple pies.

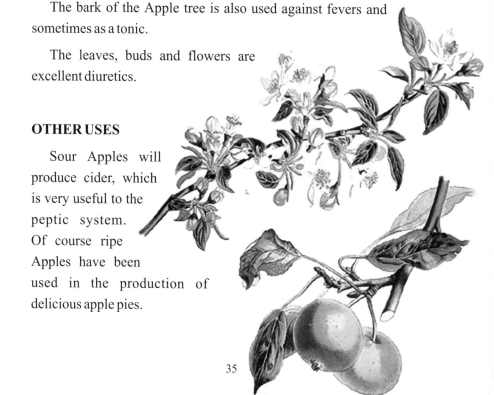

## PREPARATION AND DOSAGE

Poultice used for relieving sore eyes: Boil some very ripe Apples and mash them into poultice. Use it hot on the eyes.

Infusion: put three handfuls of flowers or buds or leaves or a combination of all of them in a liter of water and leave them soak for 3-4 hours. Drink 2-3 cups per day as a diuretic helpful for kidney stones, problems of the cyst and nephritis.

A very easy and healthful remedy provides a way to detoxify your body: for two days eat only Apples and drink Apple juice and water only. Nothing else. This will clean your stomach and intestines and relieve your liver and kidneys.

## SIDE EFFECTS

Apple kernels should be avoided because they are poisonous in large quantities. Anyway, they have a bitter taste.

## HISTORY

There is no doubt that Apple was esteemed both for its nutritional as well as for its therapeutic properties from the ancient times. Old sayings like the one in the beginning of this article are found almost everywhere around the world. Another characteristic old saying says:

" To eat an Apple going to bed

Will make the doctor begging for bread".

Such sayings remind us of the belief of the people that Apple was a cure-all fruit. This is also confirmed by a lot of ancient writers and physicians including Pliny and Dioscourides.

# Arbutus (Strawberry tree)

*Soothing, astringent, coagulant, antiseptic*

**Scientific Name:** Arbutus unede of the Ericaceae family.

**Parts Used:** leaves and fruit.

**USES:** Arbutus is used for the treatment of:

- Inflammations
- Womb hemorrhage
- Infections
- Constipation

Arbutus is used internally for soothing inflammations of the urinary system (cystitis, prostate hypertrophy, gonorrhea) and various chronic diseases of the cyst.

It is used to stop bleeding and as such is recommended for womb hemorrhage.

It is very effective for inflammations caused by gallstones and also used for dysentery and difficulties in urination.

The ripe fruit of Arbutus may be used for constipation and flatulence due to its property to expand the intestines.

## OTHER USES

A brandy produced from the Arbutus fruits is used for flu (drink or massage) when mixed with cinnamon and a little honey because it causes overheating, perspiration and drop of the fever.

## PREPARATION AND DOSAGE

Decoction: place a handful of Arbutus leaves or fruit in a liter of water. Boil them for ten minutes and leave them soaking for another fifteen minutes. We have to drink the decoction during the next 24 hours. In cases of cystitis we boil two teaspoons of Arbutus leaves in a cup of

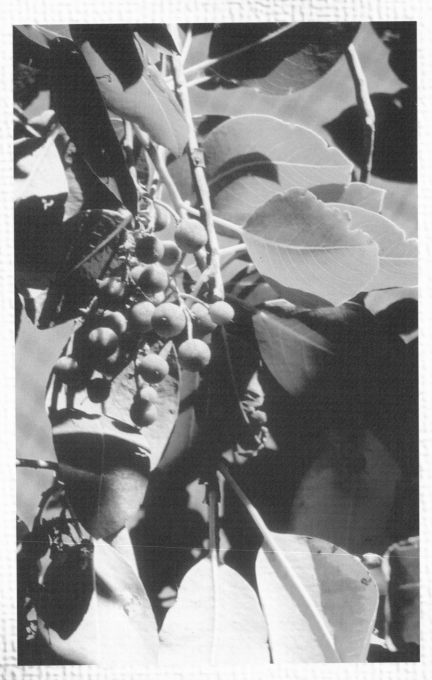

**Arbutus (strawberry tree)**     38

water for fifteen minutes and we drink two of these cups per day.

Tonic: put some Arbutus fruits in a liter of wine and add one cup of water in which we have previously heated some cinnamon and sugar.

## SIDE EFFECTS

If the decoction is taken for a long period it may cause vomiting and nausea. In cases of cystitis, a doctor should be always advised.

## HISTORY

Arbutus is common to the Mediterranean countries and the fruit was known to the ancients but according to Pliny (who gave the name Arbutus to the plant) it was not of high esteem to them. The name unede means un ede (one I eat) and this is explained by the unpalatable taste of the fruit which made every one eating them for the first time to try them again. It was mentioned though by some ancient writers that the fruits were used for food in certain cases.

# Artichoke

*Diuretic, Χολαγωγικό, appetizer*

**Scientific Name:** Cynara scolymus of the Compositae family.

**Parts Used:** Leaves

**USES:** Artichoke is used for the treatment of:
- Anorexia
- Liver
- Gall Bladder
- Cholesterol

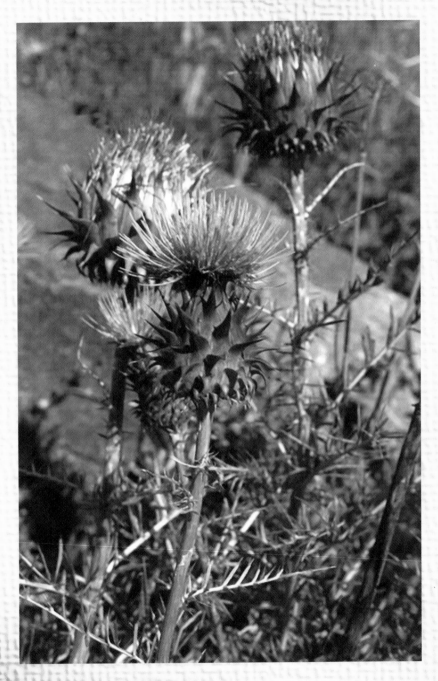

**Artichoke**

Artichoke can reduce the sugar and cholesterol levels in the blood.

Liver - it protects the liver from toxins and infections and will also strengthen its operation. It promotes liver cell formation and improves blood circulation.

Bladder - It promotes urine secretion as many as four time more than usual in a period of 12 hours.

## PREPARATION & DOSAGE

Dry Extract - the typical dosage is 5ml but not more than six grams per day. The exctract must be stored in well dosed containers away form direct sunshine and insects.

Decoction - Half cup of artichoke leaf decoction, 2-3 times daily or 3-4 ml.

## SIDE EFFECTS

Persons with a blocked bladder passage should avoid the intake of artichoke since it promotes urine secretion.

Persons with stones in the bladder should take artichoke with caution since it may provoke painful spasms.

There are reports of allergic reactions to the touch of artichoke.

## HISTORY

Artichoke was often offered as an appetizer at dinners in ancient Greece as well as ancient Rome. In modern Europe it appeared during the 15th century and has been used as a treatment for digestion problems, and for the prevention of gall bladder stone formation.

Only the dry leaves of the herb are used for medical reasons. The plant's root does not contain most of the active ingredients that have curative properties.

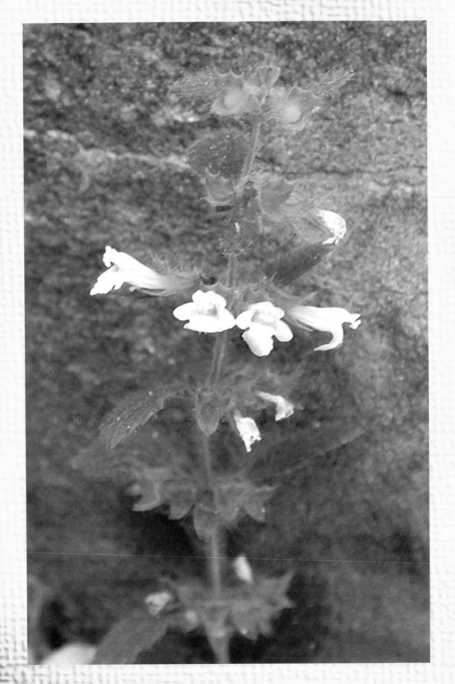

**Balm**

42

# Balm

*Tonic, sedative, calmative, diaphoretic,*
*antispasmodic, emmenagogue*

**Scientific Name:** Melissa officinalis of the Labiatae family.

**Parts Used:** herb, leaves, volatile oil and polyphenols.

■**USES:** Balm is used for the treatment of:
- Allergies
- Insomnia
- Melancholy
- Nausea
- Palpitations
- Wounds
- Hypertension
- Uric acid

The crashed Balm leaves are used externally as a poultice on wounds and insects bites. Internally, it is a well known herbal tea used as a tonic to the heart and the peptic system as well as to the brain, since it has been found very helpful in cases of melancholy, amnesia and mental weakness. The same tea is used to relieve fever in colds and flu due too its property to provoke perspiration. It is also very useful to women in cases of irregular menstrual period and menstrual cramps while it is relieving from headaches and dizziness during pregnancy.

## OTHER USES

Balm is used in perfume and cosmetics production.

Adding the decoction of Balm leaves to the bath promotes the onset of menstruation.

## PREPARATION AND DOSAGE

Decoction - boil one tablespoon of Balm flowers in a cup of water for three minutes and drink three cups daily.

Infusion - soak three teaspoons of flowering tops of the herb in a cup of water for about ten minutes and drain it. Drink 2-3 cups daily for problems of the stomach or allergies or one cup just before bedtime.

Powder - 0,7-2,6 grams per dose.

Essential oil - for indigestion or peptic problems, put a few drops of the oil in a glass of water and drink it. The same oil is used internally as an antispasmodic and anodyne. Use it externally, again diluted in some water, for massages in cases of rheumatism and migraines.

## HISTORY

The scientific name of the herb is derived from the Greek word "melissa" which mean bee, due to the fact that bees are very much attracted to Balm.

Balm has been used medicinally for centuries and it was once believed that it was the "elixir of life" providing longevity to its users. It was originally used in countries of the Middle East and the Arabs as an antidepressant to relieve from melancholy and stress and as such it has been used in Europe during the Middle Ages. In fact, it is still used this way in a lot of countries around the world.

44

# Barley
*Anti-inflammatory, cleanser, tonic*

**Scientific Name:** Hordeum vulgare.

**Parts Used:** the whole herb.

**USES:** Barley is used for the treatment of:
- Arthritis
- Gastric ulcers
- Artery blockage
- Larynx problems
- Wounds, skin tumors
- Stomach disorders
- Inflammations

External use - the soothing properties of boiled Barley make it useful for wounds and skin tumors.

Arteries - it is believed that it helps to clean the arteries and the valves around the heart where fat has built up.

Inflammations - the green juice from young Barley shoots have anti-inflammatory properties and are used for arthritis and gastric ulcers.

Barley increases muscle strength and expands the muscles especially to persons who deal with weight lifting. Also, a mixture of Barley water with milk is used for soothing the stomach and the intestines when irritated.

## OTHER USES

As you might know, beer is produced from Barley, although new ways are being employed lately.

In homeopathy, a mixture of dry Barley and peas is recommended as a substitute to coffee.

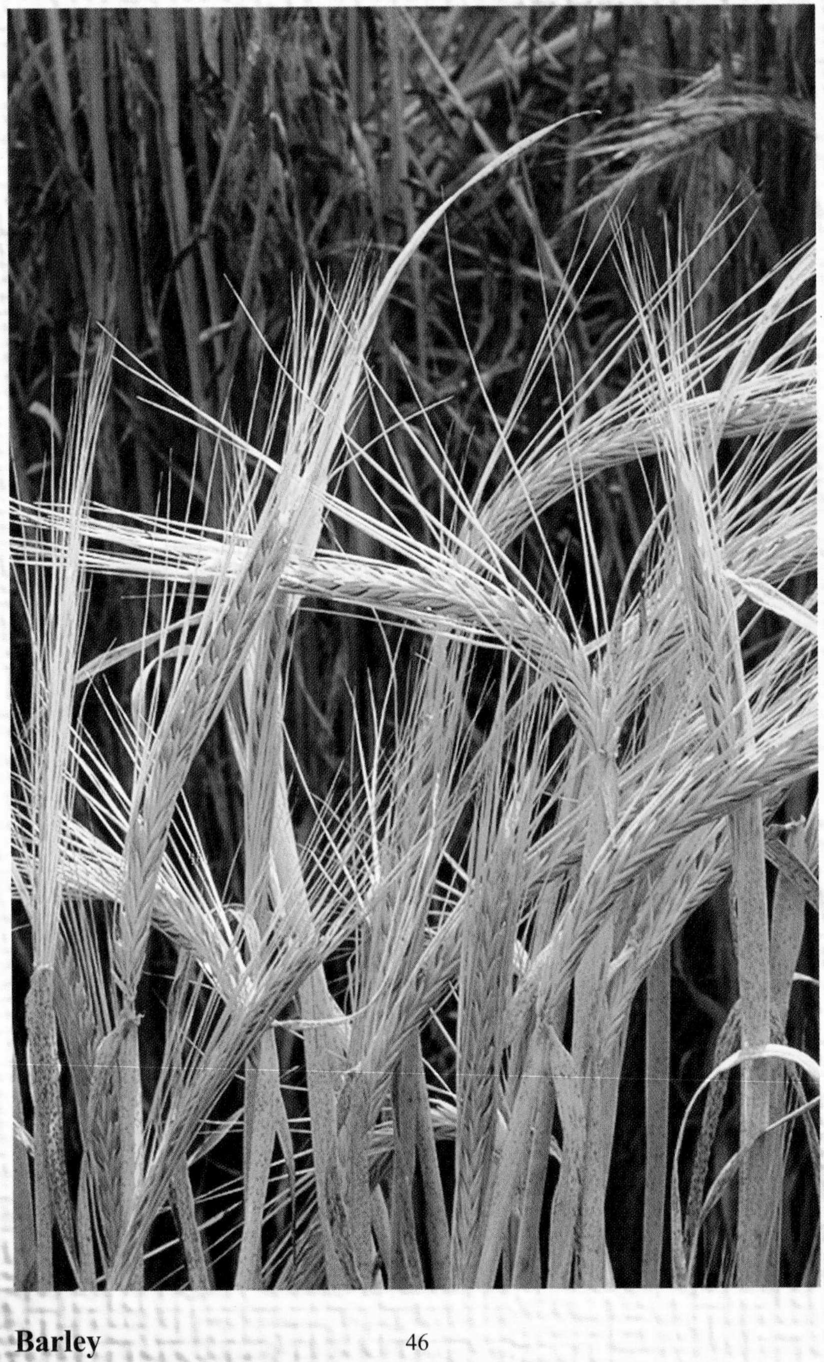

**Barley**

## PREPARATION AND DOSAGE

Decoction - wash 50 grams of Barley with water and leave it in one cup of water to soak for a few minutes. Then boil the Barley in two liters of water until the quantity of the water is reduced to half. Drain the Barley and drink the decoction, one cup at a time, three cups daily.

Barley water - wash 50 grams of Barley with cold water and then boil it in half a liter of water for 20 minutes. Drain it and drink of the infusion half a cup at a time.

## HISTORY

Barley has been cultivated for thousands of years, from the pre-ceramic period, in the Middle East area. Ancient writers mention the medicinal use of Barley in Egypt and of course its nutritional use. Ancient Egyptians used Barley as a pregnancy test. The pregnant woman was asked to spray her urine onto two bags, one containing Barley and the other one containing Wheat. If Barley shot sprigs first then this meant that the baby would be a boy and if the Wheat seeds shot first then this was a sign that the baby was a girl. In our days, research has proven the stimulating properties of pregnant' s urine on Barley seeds but did not really prove that the ancient Egyptian method was correct.

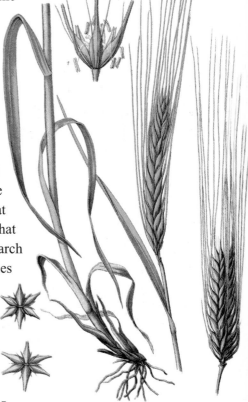

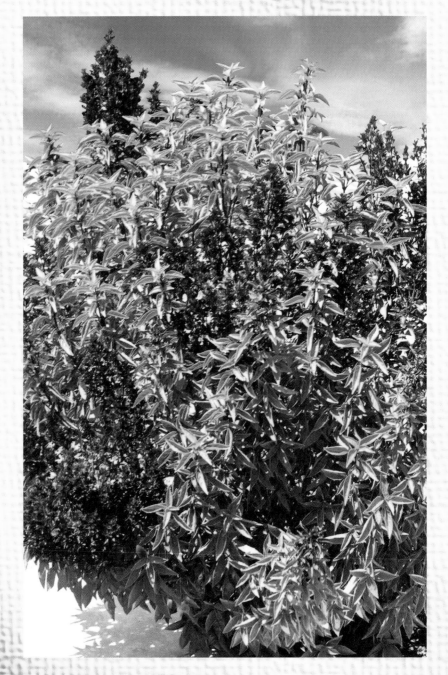

**Basil**

# Basil

*Stomachic, carminative, antispasmodic.*

**Scientific Name:** Ocimum basilicum of the Labiatae.

**Parts Used:** Leaves and branches

**USES:** Basil is used for the treatment of:
- Indigestion
- Cough
- Fever
- Dysentery
- Lung problems
- Fat accumulation
- Anxiety and depression

It is very useful and relieving in cases of stomachic and intenstine problems. It also fights vomiting, helps patients with chronic cough, and has been used for many centuries as a tranquilizer and as an antidepressant in mild cases. It is considered to be nerve tissue strengthening. Although not yet proved, there is evidence that Basil fights cancer at its initial state. If we place leaves of Basic on bee, scorpion or other insect bites, they will absorb the poisonous substances injected by the bite very quickly. In India, the herb is considered to be sacred and it will be found in almost every house. It is widely used as an antiseptic and antibacterial. Another use of the herb is to increase the production of milk during nursing.

## PREPARATION

Tea - use a tablespoon of Basil leaves in a cup of water. Leave the leaves in the hot water for 10 minutes, drain it and drink it hot. You can sweeten it with a little honey especially if it is to be used for cough. Drink one or two cups daily for most cases.

Poultice - for insect bites and external use in general, it is better to crash the leaves into poultice and apply it on the skin instead of applying the whole leaves.

Appetizer - drink half a cup of Basil tea just before each meal.

## OTHER USES

The use of Basil in cooking, is well known, especially to Italians who use it in a lot of dishes. Its strong fragrance not only freshens the air around the plant but also keeps flies and mosquitos away.

This is the reason we often see Basil plants in pots at the bedroom verandas and the house entrance in many places around the world like the Mediterranean countries and the Middle East.

## SIDE EFFECTS

Although no serious side effects have been reported in relation with Basil consumption, too much use of its tea may cause sleepiness and very rarely lack of concentration.

## HISTORY

Basil has a very rich history and has been known throughout the world. It was considered as the "Royal Herb" in France, a love symbol for the Italians and a gift from God in India. There are a lot of theories as for the derivation of its name and the most supported one says that it comes from the Greek word for king (basilias) since the ancient Greeks used the herb to freshen the air in royal palaces as well as a royal medicine. As Parkinson says, "the smell thereof is so excellent that it is fit for a King's house". Another theory says that the name is a shortened version of basilisk, a mythological creature that would kill with a look. And there are a lot of superstitions that may support this theory, like the one that connects the herb with scorpions. In fact, it is well known that scorpions often rest under the pots of Basil. During the Middle ages the Church believed that Basil was a satanic plant due to this strange attraction to scorpions. This superstition is still valid in a lot of countries. There is also a widely spread myth that if you get seduced by the alluring fragrance of Basil you eventually develop the evil characteristics of a Scorpion.

# Blackberry

*The best herb for diarrhea and dysentery but also a very good aid for hypertension.*

**Scientific Name:** Rubus fruticosus of the Rosaceae family.

**Parts Used:** leaves, berries and root.

USES: Blackberry is used as a treatment for:
- Diarrhea
- Dysentery
- Hypertension (High blood pressure)
- Hemorrhoids
- Pharyngitis
- Wound healing
- Gingivitis (inflammation of the gums)

Blackberry is a safe and gentle astringent and this is why it is used in diarrhea and dysentery. Its leaves, as well as its berries are used externally on skin rashes and wounds. It stops bleeding and relieves from the pain. The decoction of the leaves and the bark of the roots are used to treat pharyngitis and gum inflammations. The tea of Blackberry leaves will instantly reduce high blood pressure (a very good remedy for hypertensive people) while the daily consumption of this tea reduces the sugar levels in the blood of diabetic people.

## OTHER USES

Blackberries are used for the preparation of delicious sweet and sour marmalades. They are also used for the production of wine and liquer and also in a lot of children medicines, especially syrups, where the concentrated juice of Blackberries is added just to add a more attractive flavor to the medicine.

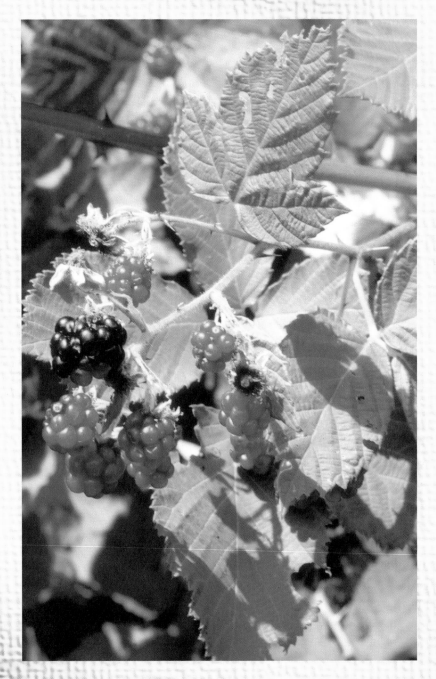

**Blackberry** 52

## PREPARATION AND DOSAGE

Tannin is one of the most useful ingredients of the root bark, the leaves and the berries of Blackberry, with more concentration in the bark of the root, than the leaves and finally the berries. Peel the bark off the root and leave it in the sun to dry. Boil 100 grams of it in 2 litres of water or milk until the fluid becomes 1 litre. You can use this decoction for diarrhea, half a cup every hour or dysentery, 1-2 cups daily. If you don't have root bark you can use 200 grams of dried leaves instead. The same decoction is used in hypertension.

Syrup - Blackberry syrup is used in pharyngitis, gum infections, as well as in hemorrhoids. You can always buy it from your local pharmacy or you can produce it by yourselves. Boil 100 grams of fresh berry juice in 50 grams of sugar until it becomes thick, uniform cream.

Externally, you can use fresh Blackberry juice on wounds and skin rashes or you can place on them fresh leaves or dry ground leaves directly.

## SIDE EFFECTS

Due to the fact that some of the ingredients of Blackberry and especially tannin may cause problems to the stomach and the intestines it is better that people who suffer from gastritis or stomach ulcers not to use Blackberry very often.

## HISTORY

The leaves of Blackberry have been used for diarrhea and dysentery for a long time. Ancient Greeks used Blackberry to treat gout while the Romans used to chew its leaves to stop the gums from bleeding. In Chinese medicine Blackberries are used as a treatment to a lot of problems. Unripe Blackberries for example are used to treat kidney problems and male impotence.

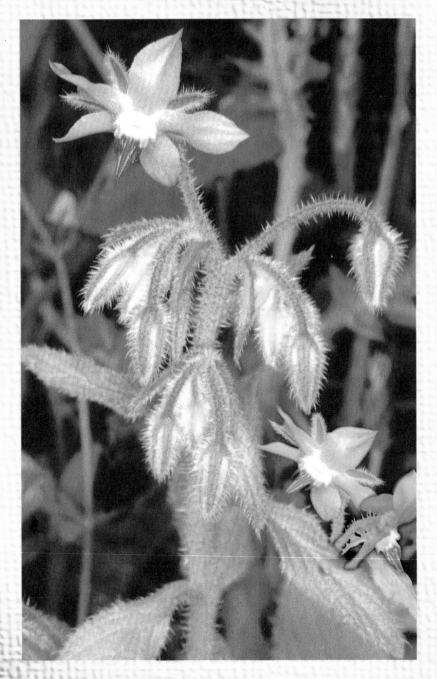

**Borage**                    54

# Borage

## Anti-inflammatory, tonic, diuretic, expectorant, galactogogue

**Scientific Name:** Borago officinalis of the Boraginaceae family.

**Parts Used:** leaves, flowers and seeds.

**USES**: Borage is used for the treatment of:
- Weakening
- Eye irritations
- Cold and fever
- Lung diseases
- Swellings

Borage restores the function of adrenalin cortex, an action very useful after a treatment with cortisone or steroids that usually weaken the adrenalin glands. It is also used for fever and during convalescence as a tonic. It has anti-inflammatory action used especially in cases of pleurisy, gall bladder and liver inflammations.

It promotes milk production in nursing women and the leaves and flowers of Borage are used for kidney stones and rheumatism.

## OTHER USES

The sugared flowers of Borage are given to patients recovering from a chronic illness as a tonic.

## PREPARATION AND DOSAGE

Infusion - put two teaspoons of dried leaves or flowers in a cup of boiling water and leave it soak for 15 minutes. Drink it three times daily for colds, bronchitis, pneumonia and fever.

Tincture - 1-4 ml, three times daily.

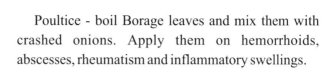

Poultice - boil Borage leaves and mix them with crashed onions. Apply them on hemorrhoids, abscesses, rheumatism and inflammatory swellings.

**SIDE EFFECTS**

Extended use of Borage is not recommended.

**HISTORY**

The scientific name Borago is believed to be derived from the Latin words Bor (heart) and "ago" (bring) revealing the tonic properties of the herb to the heart.

According to Dioscourides and Pliny, Borage was the herb that was mixed with wine and given to Eleni to forget everything. This mixture was described as Nepenthe by Homer, and it was said that it brought absolute forgetfulness to anyone drinking it. Both John Evelyn and Parkinson recommended Borage against melancholy and sorrow.

# Buckbean

*Tonic, anti-rheumatic, emetic, cholagogue, anthelmintic*

**Scientific Name:** Menyanthes trifoliata of the Menyanthaceae family.

**Parts Used:** leaves.

**USES**: Buckbean is used for the treatment of:
- Anemia
- Constipation
- Indigestion
- Bruises and wounds
- Fever
- Rheumatism

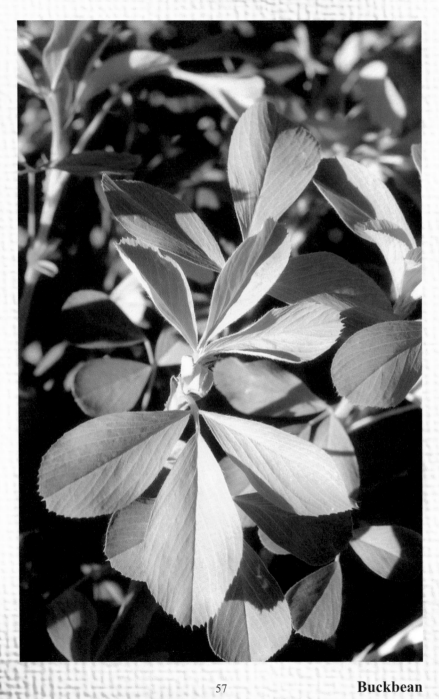

**Buckbean**

Buckbean is used externally for the treatment of glandular swellings, bruises and wounds It is very useful in the treatment of rheumatism, osteo-arthritis and rheumatoid arthritis but it should never be used for the treatment of these diseases when there is colitis or diarrhea. It is often used as a laxative because of its stimulant effect on the walls of the intestines and especially the colon.

It is used as a tonic in cases of anemia or weakness due to indigestion, liver or gall bladder problems. There are a lot of traditional remedies involving the use of Buckbean. Its juice has been effectively used for the treatment of dropsy and combined with whey it is said to cure gout. Its decoction is known to act against dyspepsia and when combined with wormwood or sage it boosts an inactive liver.

## PREPARATION AND DOSAGE

Infusion - soak 2 teaspoons of dried Buckbean leaves in a cup of hot water for 15 minutes. Drain it and drink it three times daily.

Tincture - take 1-4 ml of the tincture, three times daily.

Decoction - boil one teaspoon of dried Buckbean leaves in a cup of water for ten minutes. Drain it and drink it three times daily or use it as a compress.

Extract - the extract of the leaves of Buckbean has strong tonic properties and is very helpful in rheumatism and various skin diseases. Internally take 20 drops in some water, three times daily.

Poultice - the crashed dried leaves or the fresh leaves can be used as a poultice on bad joints, wounds, bruises and swellings.

Powder - crash the dried leaves of Buckbean into fine powder and keep them closed in a dark bottle away from sunlight. This powder is used against fever and ague and is said to be effective where other means have failed. If one tablespoon of the Buckbean powder is taken internally it acts as a good laxative.

**HISTORY**

Buckbean was considered a valuable remedy for scurvy and has been extensively used for centuries all over Europe against the disease and other problems as well as a tonic. Its scientific name Menyanthes is derived from two Greek words "minas" (month) and "anthos" (flower) describing the fact that the plant remains in flower for one month. Trifoliata clearly describes that its leaves are in threesome.

# Burning Bush
*Stomachic, sedative*

**Scientific Name:** Dictamnus albus of the Rutaceae family.

**Parts Used:** Root and leaves

USES: Burning Bush in used for the treatment of:
- Stomach disturbances
- Skin disorders
- Headache
- Toothache
- Nervous disorders

The herb is mainly used for treating disorders of the nervous system but is quite sedative for the stomach and the intestines too.

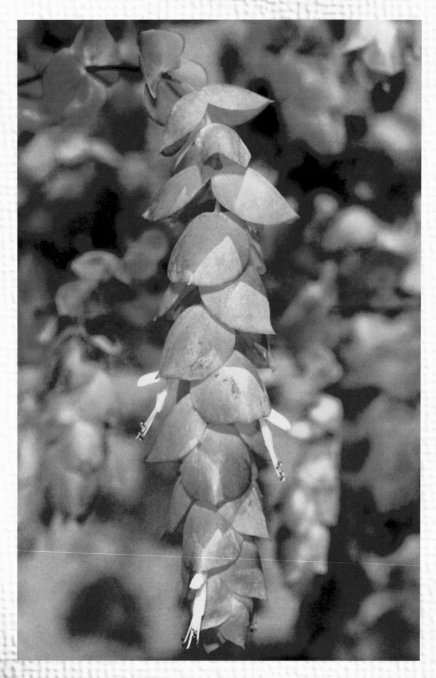

**Burning Bush** 60

## PREPARATION AND DOSAGE

Decoction - boil 10-15 grams of the root in one litre of water. Drink two cups daily.

Infusion - put 10 -15 grams of root in one litre of water and leave it for 30 minutes. To be drunk twice daily, one cup at a time.

Powder - 4 to 8 grams of powdered root, twice daily.

## OTHER USES

Burning Bush leaves have astringent properties and it is used on wounds to stop the bleeding. To do that, we grind the dried leaves until they become powder and we drop the powder directly on the wound.

Chewing the fresh leaves of the Burning Bush helps with headache and toothache and at the same time it freshens the breath.

## SIDE EFFECTS

Not recommended to pregnant women. Also, it must not be used too often because it may cause some toxic side effects.

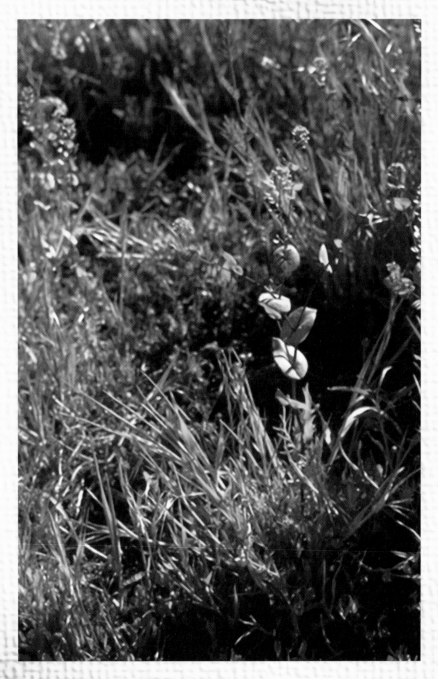

**Cardamon**

# Cardamon

*Stimulant, aromatic, digestive*

**Scientific Name:** Elettaria cardamomum of the Zingiberaceae family.
**Parts Used:** the dried, ripe seeds.

**USES:** Cardamon is used for the treatment of:
- Indigestion
- Flatulence
- Gingivitis (gum infections)

The seeds of Cardamon are used for indigestion and flatulence producing a warm but not nice feeling. Chewing the seeds have a nice taste and they are good for the gums and helpful in cases of gingivitis and mouth infections.

Externally, it is recommended to treat acme and other skin problems as well as for the treatment of hemorrhoids.

## PREPARATION AND DOSAGE

Decoction - boil 15-30 grams of Cardamon seeds in one litre of water and drink one cup every two hours.

Infusion - put two teaspoons of Cardamon seeds in a cup of hot water for ten minutes.

## SIDE EFFECTS

We must not use Cardamon daily and in general it should not be used for a period of one month during a year, because it may cause kidney problems and stomach irritation. It is also not recommended for pregnant women.

## HISTORY

It was once widely used in some European countries, especially for its stimulating properties.

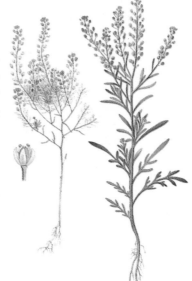

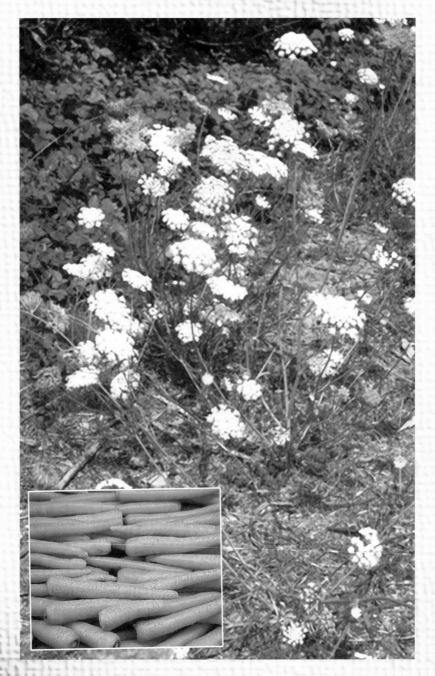

**Carrot** 64

# Carrot

*Antioxidant, diuretic, stimulant*

**Scientific Name:** Daucus carota of the Umbelliferae family.

**Parts Used:** the root (carrot), the leaves and the seeds.

**USES:** Carrot is used for the treatment of:
- Kidneys
- Tumors
- Vision
- Wounds and Burns
- Skin Protection
- Liver

It protects the skin from the Ultraviolet rays of the sun giving a nice tan to the skin. It will also make the skin shiny and will protect it from various infections. A face mask is made out of the Carrot juice that cleans the pores of the face.

Tumors: Carrots are rich in vitamins A and B which are said to have anticancer properties. Therefore Carrots are eaten preventively against the cancer of the esophagus, the lungs, the larynx, and the uterus.

Vision: it is well known that Carrots improve the vision.

Diuretic: it is very helpful to people suffering from kidney diseases and dropsy.

Its seeds are considered to be stimulants and useful in flatulence, gases of the stomach, colic, dysentery and chronic cold. In addition they are used for jaundice and for promoting menstrual period.

## OTHER USES

Carrots are used in soups, salads and several dishes. They are sometimes added in certain butters and cheeses to improve their color and taste. In Germany and France, Carrots are used for the production of a drink, since it produces more alcohol than potatoes. The residue from Carrot distillation is used as food for pigs.

## PREPARATION AND DOSAGE

Infusion - put 50 grams of the herb in one litre of hot water and leave it for ten minutes. Drink it in small wine glass doses. The infusion is used for dropsy and chronic kidney problems.

Decoction - a strong decoction is very helpful in flatulence and kidney stones.

Poultice - use the Carrot poultice on skin tumors and skin ulcers.

Carrot-soup: a very effective remedy for diarrhea. Boil 500 grams of fresh Carrots in a cup of water until they become soft. Make them into a pulp and mix them with the water in which we have boiled them.

Carrots - can be eaten raw or in several dishes. We can also use them to make Carrot juice of which we can drink two glasses daily when used for treatment.

## SIDE EFFECTS

Doctors recommend diabetics not to consume Carrot. And as with all herbs too much use is not good.

## HISTORY

Carrot has been known and used by nations and civilizations all over the world mainly for nutritional purposes. Nevertheless, Greek and Latin writers have described the medicinal use of Carrot from ancient times. Epicharmus talks about Sisaron about 500 B.C. Hippocrates uses Staphylinos about one hundred years later and Dioscourides mentions Elaphoboscum, around the 1st century A.D. The three names have been found later on to be equivalent to Carrot.

# Celery

Calming, sedative, nervine, carminative, appetizer, diuretic, stimulant, emmenagogue

**Scientific Name:** Apium graveolens of the Umbelliferae family.

**Parts Used:** seeds, leaves and roots.

**USES**: Celery is used for the treatment of:
- Arthritis
- Anorexia
- Rheumatism
- Nervousness
- Gout

The infusion of Celery is a calming aid and is used in cases of nervousness or even hysteria. It is sedative and promotes restfulness and sleep. With women it provokes the onset of menstrual period. Its juice is an excellent diuretic and is helpful in arthritis, rheumatism, dropsy, lack of appetite and gout.

## OTHER USES

Chewing seeds of Celery helps drunken persons to sober. Its consumption helps people to avoid the intake of salt and it is recommended to diabetics.

## PREPARATION AND DOSAGE

Infusion - soak 1-2 teaspoons of crashed Celery seeds in a cup of hot water for 15 minutes. Drink three cups daily.

Decoction - boil half a teaspoon of Celery seeds in half a cup of water for three minutes. Drain it and drink it three times a day.

Juice - use a vegetable juicer to extract the juice from Celery stem and leaves. Take one tablespoon of the juice 2 times a day, an hour before

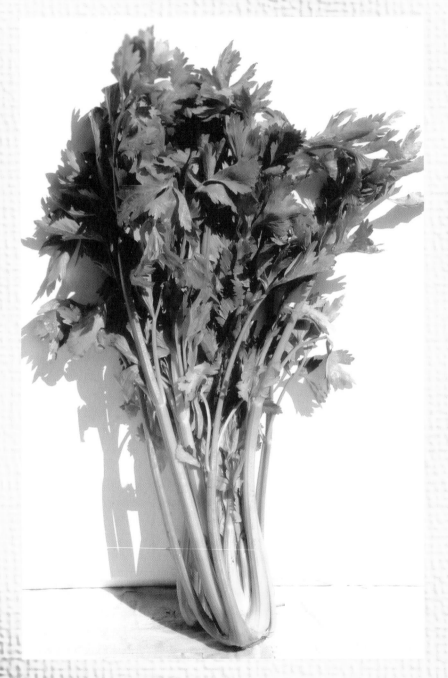

**Celery**

each meal. You can also mix the juice with Carrot or Apple juice.

Oil - take 6-8 drops of the volatile oil Apiol in a glass of water, two times daily.

Tincture - 1 to 4 ml, three times daily.

Fluid extract - 3 to 7 drops in water every 4 hours.

## SIDE EFFECTS

Celery and its juice are rich in sodium so people with High blood pressure should not exceed recommended doses.

As with all strong diuretics it is not recommended for people with severe kidney diseases although its light use is allowed.

Pregnant women should use the herb and its preparations with caution.

## HISTORY

Celery has been cultivated for more than 3,000 years in the Mediterranean area. Homer mentions its medicinal use in his books and other historians note that the herb was considered a sacred plant during the classical Hellenic era. On the other hand, the Romans used Celery more as a vegetable in their salads rather than as a medicine. They actually had some kind of superstition about it since it was believed that under certain circumstances it would bring bad lack. Today the herb is widely known all over Europe.

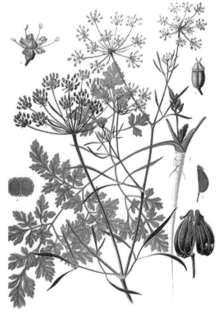

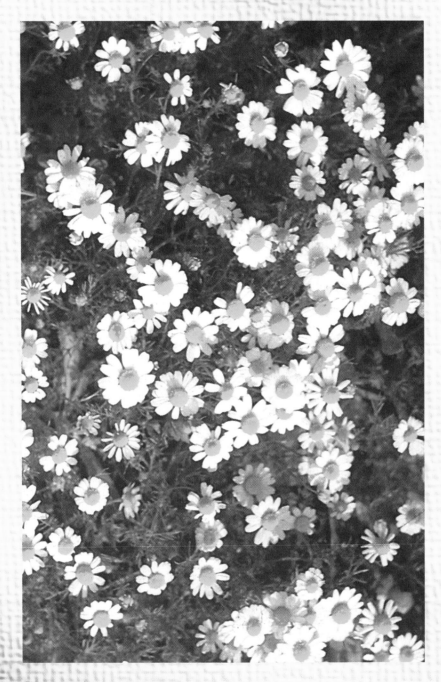

**Chamomile** 70

# Chamomile

Anti-inflammatory, antispasmodic, sedative, calmic, tonic, anodyne, stimulant, antiseptic

**Scientific Name:** Matricaria chamomilla of the Compositae family.

**Parts Used:** flowers.

USES: Chamomile is used for the treatment of:
- Mouth ulcers
- Colic
- Diarrhea
- Dyspepsia
- Sour stomach
- Skin irritations
- Eczema
- Insomnia
- Intestine irritations
- Stomach ulcers

Chamomile is used externally to promote wound and inflammation healing. Internally, Chamomile has many uses from fever and problems of the peptic system to insomnia and stress. Clinical studies have shown that Chamomile has soothing, calming properties in tea form and helps people suffering from insomnia and restless sleep. On the other hand, experiments on animals have shown that the volatile oil of Chamomile normalises the uremic function of rabbits when administered to them orally. This means that Chamomile may prove useful for the treatment of impaired kidney function. Chamomile is also widely used for its relaxing effect on the intestine muscle, which may in fact be the reason for its sedative properties in insomnia and stressful conditions.

Chamomile has been proven useful in reducing arthritic joint inflammations. It is also used externally to wash irritated eyes and cure other problems like inflammation of the eye membrane. It is used preventively for stomach ulcers but also for their treatment. In women, its antispasmodic action calms menstrual cramps and reduces the risk of premature labor. It also provokes the onset of menstruation.

In general, Chamomile boosts the infection fighting action of the white cells, stimulating the immune system.

The volatile oil of Chamomile reduces healing time of burns and wounds and the herb has been used to fight the bacteria that cause vaginal infections and was also found to induce polio virus.

## OTHER USES

Chamomile is used for the production of herbal beer. Its volatile oil is used as a tonic that revives the natural brightness of hair. It is also used in the bath for relaxation and soothing of arthritic pains. Just boil a handful of Chamomile flowers in two litres of water and mix it with the bath water.

## PREPARATION AND DOSAGE

Tea - it is very easily prepared: use 20 grams of Chamomile flowers for one litre of water. Heat the water to boiling temperature and put the flowers to soak in it for 5 to 20 minutes depending on the strength we want the tea to have. Drink it hot, 2 to 3 cups of it per day.

For massages - soak fresh or dried flowers in olive oil for 24 hours. Drain the flowers and use the oil for massaging the infected area.

Pills - Chamomile can be found in pill and tablet forms. Use 2-3 grams daily.

## SIDE EFFECTS

Although very rare, there have been reported allergic reactions to Chamomile. People allergic to plants of the Asteraceae family must avoid the use of Chamomile. It can be safely used during pregnancy and nursing.

The very frequent use of Chamomile may cause nausea, dizziness and vomiting.

## HISTORY

Chamomile is being used for centuries mainly for the treatment of problems of the peptic system. In ancient Egypt it was dedicated to the God of the sun due to its curative properties. Its tea is drunk in a lot of places around the world and it is esteemed for its healing action on the kidneys and the spleen. For thousands of years, Chamomile has been used as a natural tranquilizer for problems of the nervous system, stress and insomnia.

The fresh plant has an intense apple scent, a fact that gave the Greek name to the plant "Chamomile" meaning apple of the earth. Similarly, the Spanish named it "Manzanilla" meaning small apple.

# Cherry tree
*Diuretic, astringent*

**Scientific Name:** Prunus cerasus of the Rosaceae family.

**Parts Used:** leaves, fruit and stalk.

**USES:** Cherry tree is used for the treatment of:
- Bronchitis
- Asthma
- Cough
- Diabetes
- Cocitis
- Eye irritation

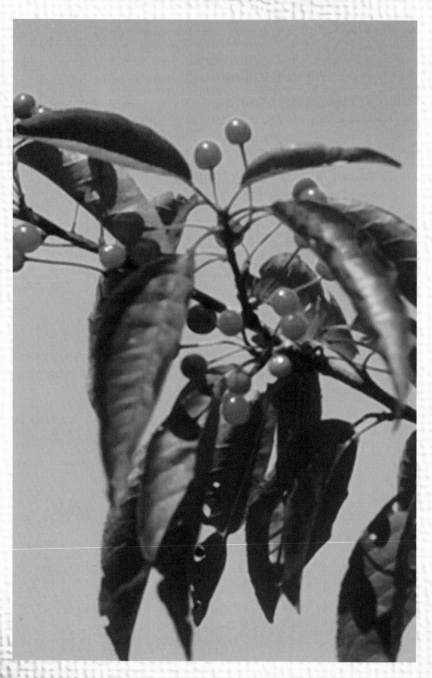

**Cherry tree**

Cherry tree is basically used for the treatment of irritated throat to people suffering from cough, bronchitis and cocitis. It helps in the stabilization of asthma in combination with other herbs. It has shown digestive properties and is used in cases of indigestion and dyspepsia. Externally, it is used to wash the eyes in cases of irritation.

## OTHER USES

Traditional herbal medicine recommends cherry tree for the treatment of rapid, weak circulation, continual irritating cough, cardiac palpitations from debility, loss of appetite as well as for cardiac pain. It is safely recommended to people suffering from heart diseases because it is rich in sugars that are being easily metabolized.

## PREPARATION AND DOSAGE

Decoction - cut the dry stalks of Cherry tree in fine pieces, put them in water and leave them for one day to soften. Boil one handful of them in one litre of water for ten minutes and drink 3-4 cups daily.

Infusion - put one teaspoon of finely cut leaves and stalks in a cup of hot water and leave them soaking for 10-15 minutes. Drink 3 cups daily.

Bath - use one handful of dried leaves and stalks for every liter of water.

Tincture - take 1-2 ml of the tincture three times per day.

## SIDE EFFECTS

Although in theory very large amounts of cherry pose the risk of causing cyanide poisoning, no such incidence has ever been reported making the herb safe for use.

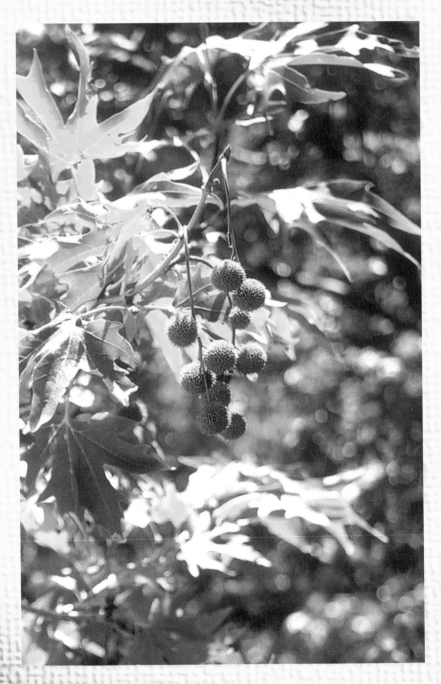

**Chessnut tree**

# Chestnut tree
*Anti-inflammatory, tonic*

**Scientific Name:** Aesculus hippocastanum of the Sapindaceae family.

**Parts Used:** leaves, fruit and bark.

**USES:** Chestnut tree is used for the treatment of:
- Hemorrhoids
- Arthritis
- Diarrhea
- Tumors
- Wounds
- Varicose veins
- Fever

Chestnuts are widely used in Europe for their anti-inflammatory properties as well as for the treatment of various vein problems. They are used especially for varicose veins, leg inflammations and diarrhea. It also fights tumors and its leaves and bark are used for fever conditions.

## OTHER USES

Chestnuts are used for the production of excellent jams and sweets.

In some Eastern European countries, Chestnuts are used to feed horses and cows who eat them with great pleasure contrary to pigs that do not even touch them.

## PREPARATION AND DOSAGE

Decoction - boil one handful of the bark or the leaves in one litre of water for ten minutes and then drain them. You can drink

2-3 cups daily of this decoction which is very useful for washing infected eyes, as an appetizer, tonic and digestive aid.

Infusion - put 30 grams of leaves in a cup of hot water and leave them soak for 10 minutes before draining. Drink one tablespoon to one cup at a time, according to the disease, three times daily.

Poultice - boil some Chestnut leaves and apply them on hemorrhoids.

It is recommended to use only standardized extracts internally.

## SIDE EFFECTS

People suffering from liver or kidney diseases should avoid Chestnuts in general unless recommended by their doctor.

## HISTORY

The leaves of the Chestnut tree have been used in the past and in traditional medicine against fevers and cough and to relieve from the pains of arthritis and rheumatism. A poultice from the fruit was used in the past to heal skin ulcers and cancers and for the treatment of varicose veins.

# Chicory

## Tonic, stomachic, diuretic, cholagogue, expectorant

**Scientific Name:** Cichorium intybus of the Compositae family.

**Parts Used:** flowering herb and roots.

**USES:** Chicory is used for the treatment of:
- Gastritis
- Constipation
- Jaundice
- Liver
- Spleen
- Indigestion
- Poor appetite

Studies performed by Arullani (1937) and Ploese (1940) have proven that the juice of Chicory leaves have anti-diabetic properties. In 1982, Said mentions in his book "Diseases of the liver: Greco-Arab concepts" that Chicory has anti-inflammatory and anti-asthmatic properties and that in the Arab and Greek traditional medicine Chicory sperms were used in certain remedies to cure liver and gall diseases. Following this report, researchers performed experiments which proved that the methanolic extract from Chicory sperms has protective action on the liver.

Chicory is often recommended for jaundice, gall bladder problems and constipation. The juice of the leaves and tea produced from the flowering herb promote urine production, gallstone dilution and fights internal inflammations. It is also very useful for gastritis and digestion problems.

### OTHER USES

The roots of Chicory are used as a coffee substitute after they are processed in a special way (café de chicoree, sucory).

Chicory leaves are used in blue paint.

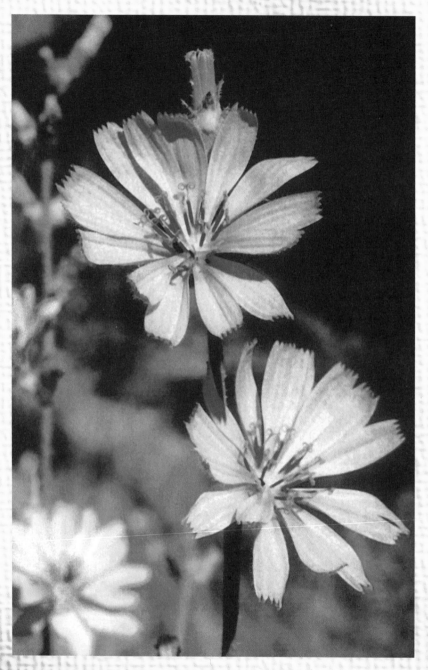

**Chicory**

## PREPARATION AND DOSAGE

Decoction - boil one tablespoon of the root or the leaves of Chicory in half a cup of water for ten minutes. Drain it and drink it, one mouthful at a time, one to one and a half cups per day maximum. It is very good for glandular and peptic problems.

Juice - one tablespoon in a cup of water or milk, three times a day.

Distilled water - soak some Chicory flowers in distilled water for twenty minutes and apply it on the eyes to relieve from irritation.

Poultice - boil the leaves of Chicory, put them in a piece of cloth and apply them on the affected area. It relieves from painful inflammations.

## SIDE EFFECTS

There has been no poisoning report from eating Chicory but it is better not to eat bitter Chicory very often because it may cause problems to the peptic system.

Prolonged use of Chicory may cause vision problems.

## HISTORY

Chicory is one of the oldest herbs and it is even mentioned in Ebers papyrus which was written around 4,000 B.C. It is mentioned by a lot of historians including Theophrastus, Pliny and Dioscourides who used the name Chicorion or Chicory.

Its scientific name Chicorium intybus is derived from the Greek word "kihora" and the Latin word "intubus". In ancient Rome, Chicory was eaten raw in the salad.

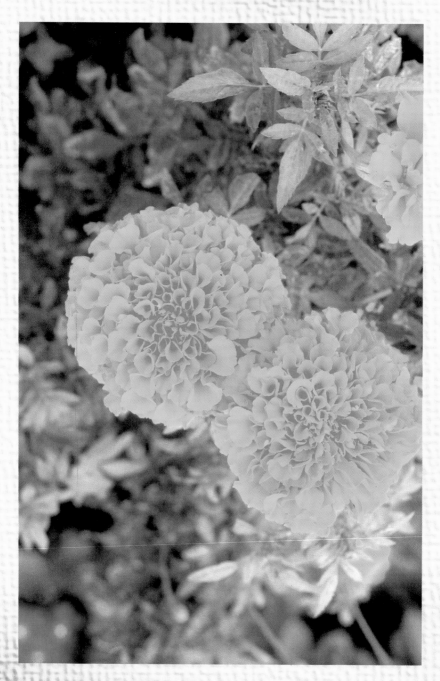

**Chrysanthemum**

# Chrysanthemum
Anti-inflammatory, antipyretic,
reduces high blood pressure

**Scientific Name:**
Chrysanthemum vulgare of the
Morifolium family.

**Parts Used:** flowers and roots.

USES: Chrysanthemum is used for
the treatment of:
- Rheumatism
- Neuralgias
- Headache
- Confusion

The volatile oil of Chrysanthemum is used externally for local massages in cases of rheumatism. The infusion of its root is used in gargles for partial paralysis of the tongue or the lips. People suffering from chronic rheumatism or head neuralgias will be benefited if they chew Chrysanthemum root every day for several months. It soothes the stomach and improves vision while it has been found very helpful in cases of dizziness and confusion. It reduces high blood pressure, relieves from headaches and is used in common cold and fever.

## PREPARATION AND DOSAGE
Infusion - soak two teaspoons of Chrysanthemum flowers in one cup of fresh water for one hour. Sweeten the infusion with some honey and drink three cups daily.

We can also buy Chrysanthemum powder or its volatile oil from the market.

## SIDE EFFECTS
People suffering from weakness or diarrhea should avoid the use of Chrysanthemum.

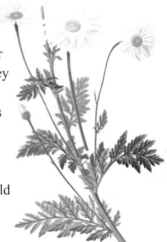

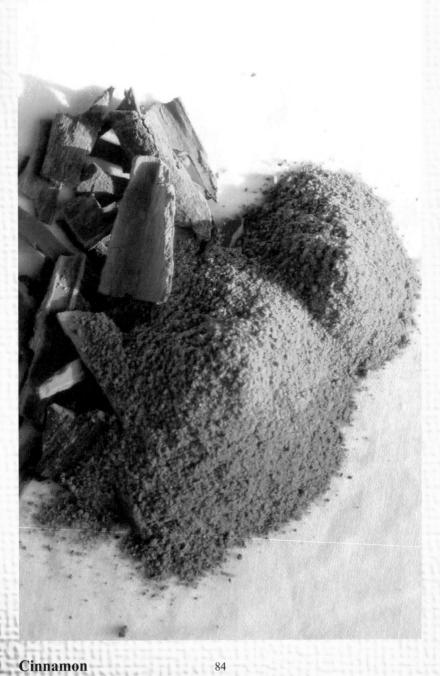

**Cinnamon** 84

# Cinnamon

*Analgesic, antiseptic, anti-rheumatic, aromatic,*
*antispasmodic, diuretic, sedative, aphrodisiac*

**Scientific Name:**
Cinnamonum zeylanicum of
the Lauraceae family.

**Parts Used:** the dried bark and
its volatile oil.

**USES:** Cinnamon is used for the
treatment of:

- Respiratory problems
- Bronchitis
- Hyperemia
- Diarrhea
- Dysentery
- Liver problems
- Kidneys
- Melancholy
- Swelling

It is recommended in cases of fatigue and weakness due to its tonic properties and the fact that it stimulates the respiratory circulation. It is used internally to stop diarrhea and spasms of the stomach and the intestines. Externally, it may be used in cases of psoriasis, skin rashes, insect and even snakebites. It is also very relieving in menstrual pains but it is suspected to discontinue pregnancy. It is of course known to be an aphrodisiac and helps with male impotence.

## PREPARATION AND DOSAGE

Decoction - boil 10 grams of the Cinnamon bark in one litre of water and drink of it whenever you like.

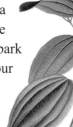

Tea - you can combine cinnamon with any tea you want. Just place a small piece of the bark in the water to be used for tea and boil the water with the bark in it. It will add a pleasant smell and flavor to your tea.

A flu remedy - put one piece of Cinnamon bark in a cup of water together with a dried clover bud and boil them for 20 minutes. Drain it, add one tablespoon of honey and half a cup fresh lemon juice. Drink this hot and it will relieve you from the flu symptoms.

## OTHER USES

Cinnamon is used in many countries as a spice and aromatic in cooking and cakes.

## SIDE EFFECTS

Be careful when using Cinnamon volatile oil externally because it may cause local leucodermia (white skin).

# Cleavers

*Cleanser, antispasmodic, diuretic, perspiratory*

**Scientific Name:** Galium aparine of the Rubiacecae family.

**Parts Used:** the whole plant.

USES: Cleavers is used for the treatment of:
- Insomnia
- Hemorrhage
- Skin infections
- Ulcers
- Wounds and sores
- Measles
- Intestine and stomach colds
- Freckles

Cleavers is mainly used externally, for the treatment of skin sores and wounds, acme, freckles, ulcers and even snakebites. It is though used also internally for the treatment of intestine and stomach colds, measles

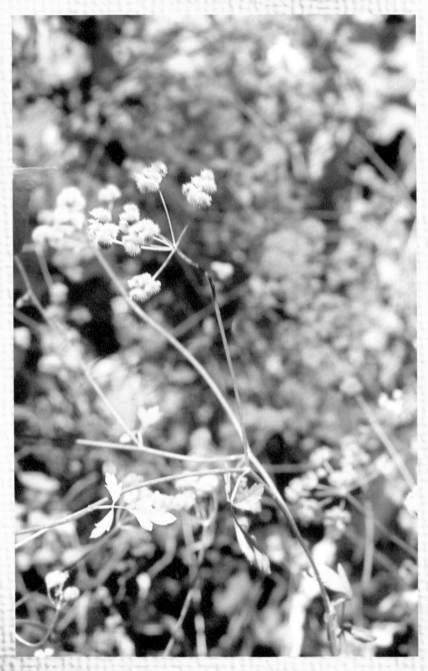

87 **Cleavers**

and insomnia.

## OTHER USES

Use the juice of the herb or dry it for later use. The decoction or the infusion of the dried herb is widely used for skin infections. The juice or the infusion of the herb must be applied daily and allowed to dry. Before the application, clean the wound or the infected area with a piece of cloth soaked in alcohol. The crushed and dry leaves of Cleavers can be applied directly on the wound to stop bleeding.

## PREPARATION AND DOSAGE

Decoction - boil 40 grams of the fresh roots of Cleavers in one litre of water for ten minutes. In cases of measles drink one teaspoon of this every five minutes. For gallstones we can drink three cups daily. The same decoction is used to eliminate freckles and in cases of sunburn. Just use a piece of cloth or sponge to soak in the decoction to apply it to the face.

Infusion - soak 30 grams of the herb in half litre of hot water for two hours. Take 2-8 teaspoons, four times daily.

Tincture - take 20-30 drops of it three times daily.

Salve - you can prepare a salve by mixing the fresh juice of Cleavers with butter, to use it on skin infections. When applied, renew the salve every three hours.

Juice - the juice is recommended in doses of 3 ounces, twice daily. It is given in cases of dropsical complaints, as it operates with significant power on the urinary secretion and the urinary organs. It is also given in cases of obstruction of these organs as it acts as a solvent of stones in the bladder.

## SIDE EFFECTS

The high level of tannin contained in Cleavers makes it very astringent, therefore it should not be used continuously. Take it for two weeks, make a break of one or two weeks and then use it again.

The juice is a rather powerful diuretic. Therefore it is not recommended to people with a tendency for diabetes.

## HISTORY

Most of the local names of Cleavers are connected with its clinging property. Its medicinal use is first mentioned by the Greeks, who named the herb "Philanthropon" meaning "friend of man" which was later on Anglicized to "Loveman". Dioscourides mentions that Greek shepherds used the stems of the herb to make a rough sieve and similarly Linnaeus mentions the same use being made in Sweden in the country districts.

# Clove
*Antiseptic, antispasmodic, aphrodisiac, calming, digestive.*

**Scientific Name:** Eugenia aromatica of the Myrtaceae family.

**Parts Used:** Flower buds (or undeveloped flowers)

**USES:** Clove is used for the treatment of:
- Toothache
- Male impotency
- Gastritis
- Cholera
- Arthritis

External use - Clove oil is used as an oral anesthetic by dentists and to disinfect root canals. It also relieves from toothache, arthritis, muscle pains and wound pain.

Internally - Clove is chewed (in its dried form) to increase male potency. It is also very useful for indigestion, nausea, vomiting and other

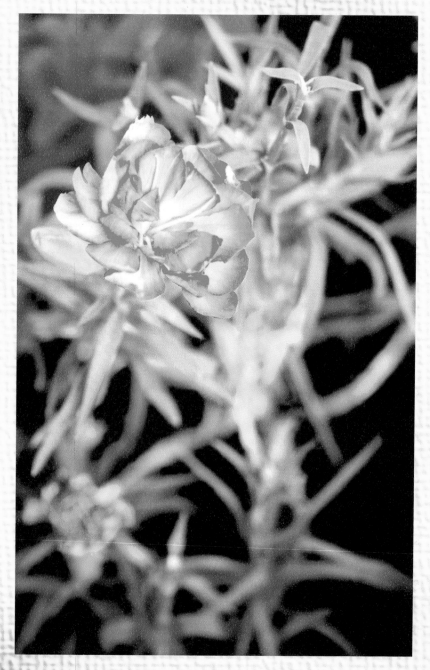

**Clove**

digestive problems.

## PREPARATIONS AND DOSAGE

Decoction - Boil one teaspoon of Clove in powder form for about 10 minutes in one cup of water. Cover the cup for another 10 minutes (or until it cools down) and drink it. You can have three cups daily. Be careful not to give this decoction to children under 2 years of age. It is recommended to give a "lighter" tea to bigger children or old people.

Clove oil - Clove oil is used to temporarily relieve toothache. Just put some Clove oil onto a piece of cotton swab and place it directly on the aching tooth. Or apply directly a drop of Clove oil into the tooth cavity.

Gargles - put one drop of Clove oil into half a glass of water and gargle with it to freshen your month and breath. The dilution is better not to be swallowed. As an alternative, we can boil some clove buds and store the decoction in a bottle to be used for gargles whenever needed.

Bath put a few drops of Clove oil in the water and relax in your bath for 15 minutes. This relieves from arthritis and back pains.

## OTHER USES

Clove oil in often used in the production of cosmetics, soaps and fragrances and to add flavor in a variety of medicines and dental items.

Dried Clove is used as a spice in cooking especially in some Asian countries although its use in the kitchen has now spread around the world.

Another practical use is as insect repellant. If you pinch an apple with some Clove buds it will keep flies and mosquitos away.

## SIDE EFFECTS

Clove oil should not be taken orally too often, that is why it is not recommended to give it to small children because they may not

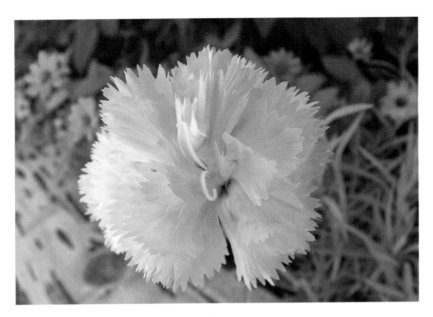

understand that they must not swallow it.

Clove oil may develop a rash when used externally so it is better to dilute it before using it directly on the skin. Its use is not recommended to pregnant and nursing women.

## HISTORY

Although Clove was imported in Europe around the 4th century A.D., its use was widely spread only after the middle ages, when it was given to patients with diarrhea, stomach problems, worms, nausea, vomiting and even infertility. It was also used to relieve from toothache. Still, the use of Clove goes back to the 3rd century B.C. when the Chinese were using it to treat indigestion, diarrhea, fungal infections like athlete's foot and of course bad breath. During the Han Dynasty (207 B.C. to 220 A.D.) all Chinese appearing to the emperor were forced to chew Clove buds to improve their bad breath. In some other places, people used to make necklaces out of Clove buds because they thought they keep illnesses away.

# Coriander

*Stimulant, antispasmodic,*
*aromatic aphrodisiac, digestive*

**Scientific Name:** Coriandrum sativum of the Umbelliferae family.

**Parts Used:** seeds and flowers.

**USES:** Coriander is used for the treatment of:
- Stomach pains
- Flatulence
- Nervous Anorexia
- Weakness
- Rheumatism
- Headaches

Coriander is used externally for rheumatism and to sooth pains in the joints. It is also made into salve to be used on irritated eyes.

Internally, it is used for headaches, skin rashes, urinary problems, sore throat and high fever.

The Chinese traditional medicine recommends Coriander seeds for stomach pain, dyspepsia and anorexia. They also use the seeds as well as the leaves as body and mouth aromatic.

The oil of Coriander is also useful for colic pain, neuralgias and rheumatism while it is considered to have antibacterial properties.


## OTHER USES

Coriander seeds are used as a spice and also in beer production as an aromatic. A big number of beverages include Coriander and its flavor is also used in the production of medicines.


## PREPARATION AND DOSAGE

Decoction - Boil one teaspoon of Coriander seeds in a cup of water for

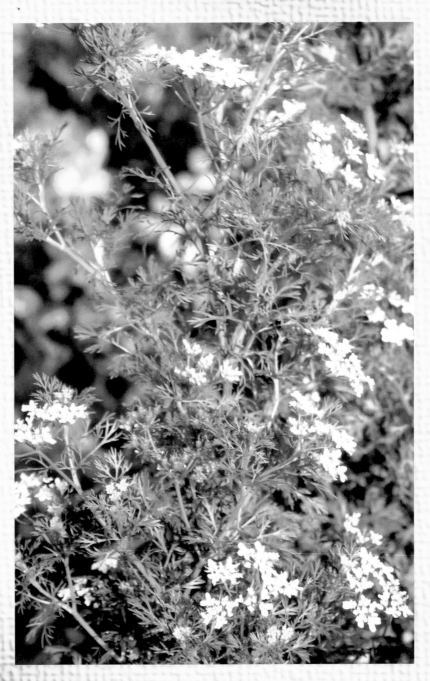

**Coriander**

ten minutes. Drain it and drink one cup after each meal.

Infusion - put two teaspoons of the seeds in a cup of hot water. Soak them for 20 minutes, drain it and drink one cup per day.

Dilution - dilute a quarter to half a teaspoon of Coriander seed powder in one cup of water and drink it.

Tincture - we can find Coriander tincture at the pharmacy. Use 10-20 drops after each meal.

Volatile oil - use 2-3 drops of the oil, combined with honey, three times daily after each meal.

Salve - we can find it at the pharmacies and is used externally to sooth rheumatic pains.

**SIDE EFFECTS**

Extreme use of Coriander may cause problems to the nervous system.

**HISTORY**

Coriander was esteemed for its aromatic and medicinal properties from ancient times and this might be the reason why it is used in almost every part of the world. It is believed that it was cultivated in Babylonia gardens. During the Middle Ages it was found in almost all kitchens in Europe and was used as a meat preservative in combination with vinegar as well as a spice. They used to prepare aphrodisiac drinks with it but also madicines for the cure of acme in adults. Today it grows freely in all Mediterranean countries but is also cultivated in other parts of the world as well, because of its wide use.

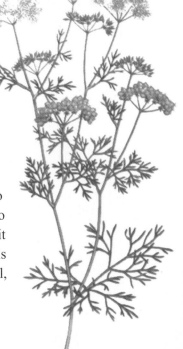

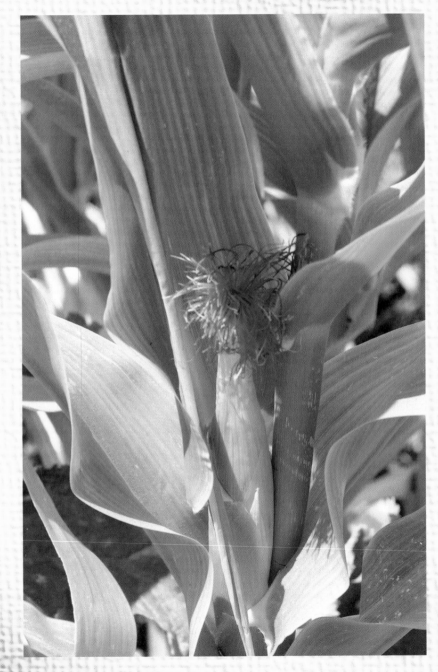

**Corn**

# Corn

*Diuretic, light tonic, anti-inflammatory*

**Scientific Name:** Zea mays of the Graminaceae family.

**Parts Used:** The "hair" of corn (the thin fibers that develop around the seeds).

**USES:** Corn is used for the treatment of:
- Inflammations
- Kidney stones
- Urethra Infections
- Cystitis (bladder disease)
- Prostate
- Rheumatism
- Ulcer

## PREPARATION AND DOSAGE

Infusion - put two teaspoons of dried Corn fibers in a cup of hot water and cover it for 15 minutes. Drink one cup, three times daily.

It is better to gather the fibers while they are still fresh on the Corn because when they dry up on the corn they loose their properties. After we gather them, we can dry them in the sun. An alternative to the fibers, is the seed of the corn which is not the same effective though. Instead of the fibers, use the same quantity of crashed (not powdered) corn seeds.

## OTHER USES

Corn is widely cultivated all over the world and people have developed a lot of uses with it. The well known cornflakes are very nourishing and are also recommended to people suffering from constipation. In many places around the world, the corn flour is used extensively for the production of bread, which is in fact more nourishing than wheat bread and is considered helpful to people with kidney and liver problems.

In Mexico, Corn is being used for the production of liqueurs and other alcoholic drinks, even for the brewing of beer. The Mexican "Pulgue de Mahis" is one of these liqueurs and is exported to the whole world.

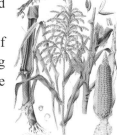

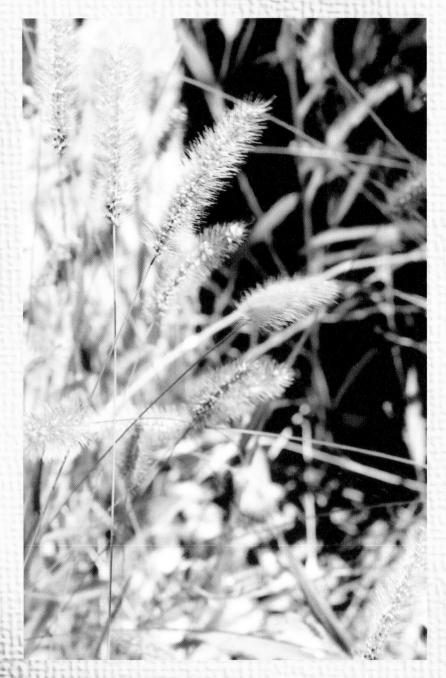

**Couchgrass** 98

# Couchgrass

*Diuretic and very helpful in problems of the uric system.*

**Scientific Name:** Agropyron repens of the Graminaceae family.

**Parts Used:** Root

**USES:** Couchgrass is used for the treatment of:
- Cystitis
- Urethritis
- Prostate
- Inflammation
- Gall Bladder stones
- Jaundice

Couchgrass has been proven very effective in various problems of the uric system. In cases of infections of the uric system it will calm the irritation and is very sedative in cases of gall bladder stones. It is assumed that its diuretic effect is derived from the sugar it contains.

## PREPARATION AND DOSAGE

Tea - use two teaspoons of the dried root of Couchgrass in one cup of water. We boil it for about 10 minutes and we drink it three times daily.

Tincture - instead of tea, we can drink 2-4 ml of the tincture of Couchgrass again three times daily.

## OTHER USES

Another name of Couchgrass is dog grass which is derived from its property to cure the dogs when they are sick. Sometimes we can see dogs chewing Couchgrass even if the are not vegetarian, just because the grass has the tendency to irritate their throat, provoking vomiting.

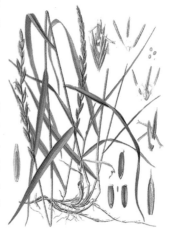

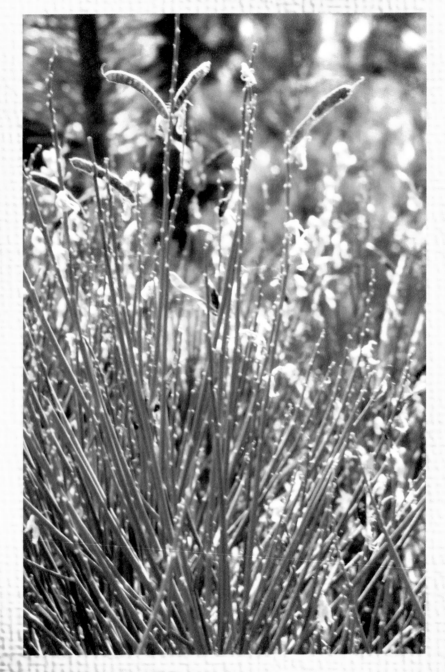

**Cumin**

# Cumin

Heart tonic, diuretic, emmenagogue,
antispasmodic, expectorant, antipyretic

**Scientific Name:** Cuminum cyminum of the Umbeliferae family.

**Parts Used:** dried seeds.

USES: Cumin is used for the treatment of:

- Flatulence
- Fever
- Palpitations
- Orchitis
- Anorexia
- Dyspepsia
- Colic

Cumin is used internally for the excess gases produced in the stomach and relieves from flatulence. It has been proven very helpful in anorexia and indigestion. It is used as a tonic for the heart, a property that also helps people suffering from palpitations.

As an emmenagogue it helps women with difficulties or abnormalities in their menstrual cycle. It also increases milk production in nursing women.

It is a valuable antispasmodic and antipyretic (fights fever) and soothing in colic pain (especially in young children).

**OTHER USES**

Chewing Cumin seeds strengthens the peptic system and the function of the liver.

The leaves of Cumin are often used in salads.

The volatile oil is used to add flavor to drinks, ice cream, sweets, gums and bread.

## PREPARATION AND DOSAGE

Decoction - boil one teaspoon of Cumin seeds in half a cup of water for ten minutes and leave the seeds soak in the water until it is cold. Drink half a cup, three times daily.

Infusion - soak one tablespoon of Cumin seeds in a cup of hot water for ten minutes. For a stronger infusion put two or more tablespoons of seeds.

Powder - take a quarter to half a teaspoon of Cumin seeds powder in some water, three times daily.

## SIDE EFFECTS

Don't drink the decoction or the infusion of Cumin seeds for more than four consecutive days because it may cause dizziness.

## HISTORY

Cumin is mentioned in the Bible and also by Hippocrates and Dioscourides who recommended its medicinal use. In ancient Greece, Cumin symbolised strong lust.

102

# Daisy
*Fights inflammations, fever and hypertension*

**Scientific Name:** Chrysanthemum leucanthemum of the Compositae family.

**Parts Used:** flowers.

USES: Daisy is used for the treatment of:
- Inflammtions
- Fever
- Hypertension
- Bad vision
- Liver infections

Daisy is recommended for the relief of the brain and the liver and for the improvement of vision. It can be used against any kind of inflammation, for fevers, even for common colds. It is especially good for high fevers accompanied by headaches. The white Daisy is used to reduce high blood pressure.

## OTHER USES

We can use the extract of Daisy externally on bruises and wounds. It is also very effective for toothache. Just chew some flowers and leave them on the tooth you feel the pain.

## PREPARATION AND DOSAGE

Decoction - boil the flowers of two daisies in a cup of water for 5 minutes. Drain the flowers and add some sugar or preferably honey to sweeten it and drink it.

Infusion - put one tablespoon of daisy flowers in a cup of boiling water and leave it for half an hour. Drink only one cup of this infusion per day.

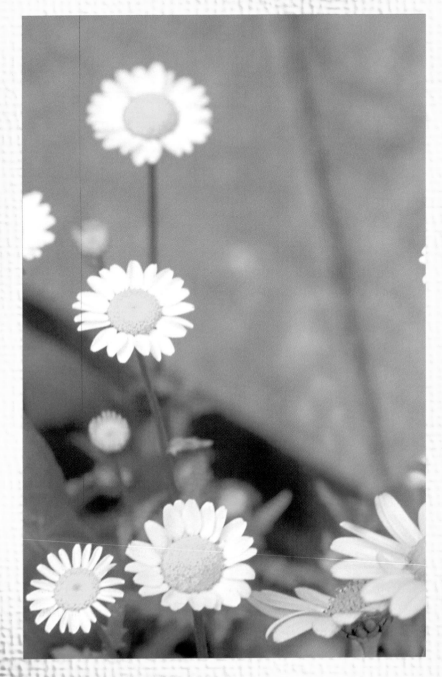

**Daisy** 104

## SIDE EFFECTS

Daisy is not recommended to people that suffer from weakness or diarrhea.

## HISTORY

The ancient Greeks thought of the flower as a woman's therapeutic herb (menstrual pains, irregular menstrual period etc) and maybe this is the reason why it was dedicated to the Goddess Artemis.

# Dill

*Aromatic, Stomachic, fights inflammations.*

**Scientific Name:** Anethum graveolens of the Umbelliferae family.

**Parts Used:** Seeds, leaves, flowers and roots.

**USES:** Dill in used as a treatment for:
- Stomach problems
- Urination problems
- Kidney stones
- Insomnia
- Kidney colic
- Indigestion

It is an excellent sedative to intestine swelling especially to children, relieving them fast and effectively even from colic pains that are sometimes produced by the swelling. Dill tea or Dill seeds in red wine have been used traditionally to calm an upset stomach. It is also used as an appetizer, it fights insomnia and has aromatic properties that offer a fresh breath.

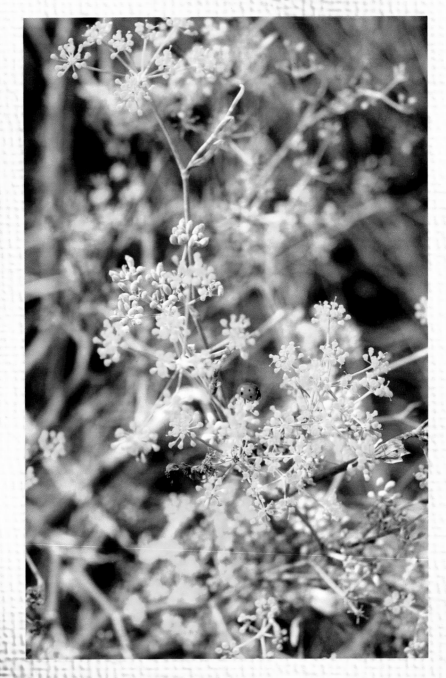

**Dill** 106

## PREPARATION AND DOSAGE

Decoction - Boil two teaspoons of Dill seeds into one litre of water for 10-15 minutes. Drain the seeds and drink half a cup of the decoction 1-2 times daily in small sips.

Dill water - Leave two handfuls of Dill in one litre of water for the whole night at room temperature. We can then drink 1-2 cups of this water daily.

## OTHER USES

We can find Dill water at the pharmacies which we can use for month gargles to fight bad breath. A very good recipe is 2-3 branches of flowered Dill in one litre of virgin oil together with a branch of Rosemary. We leave the herbs in the oil for several days and then we use it to marinate chicken or fish or even use it in salads. The oil will give them a very nice and distinctive taste.

## SIDE EFFECTS

Dill cannot be used during pregnancy because it may cause abortion. It is also suggested that the tea of the seeds of Dill should not be drunk very often because it may weaken the vision.

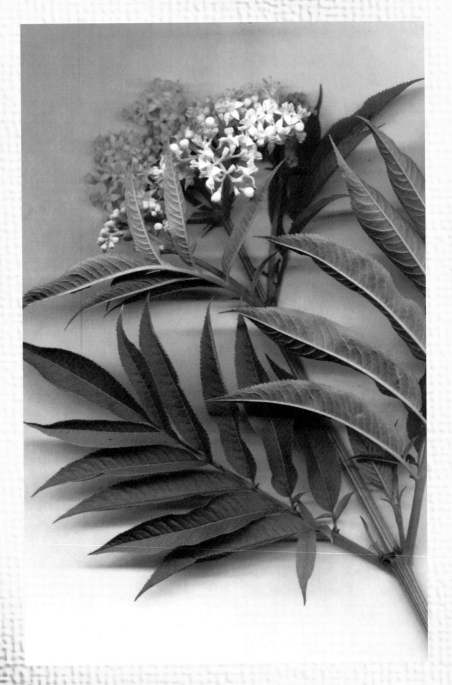

**Elder** 108

# Elder

*Tonic, diuretic, purifier, anti-inflammatory*

**Scientific Name:** Sambuccus nigra of the Caprifoliaceae family.

**Parts Used:** leaves, flowers, fruit and bark.

**USES**: Elder is used for the treatment of:

- Skin problems
- Simple herpes
- Colds
- Dry cough
- Sore throat
- Pneumonia
- Inflammations

Elder has the remarkable property to reduce skin wrinkles and soften the skin in general, when applied externally. The juice of Elder is used as a tonic to the reproductive system and various glands of the body. A tea produced from the leaves and young sprigs increases urine production and helps in expelling excess water from the blood. Black Elder is employed in the treatment of urine problems, kidney malfunction, dropsy, rheumatic diseases and constipation.

Tea from the flowers increases perspiration and is used for colds and rheumatism.

Elder jam is considered to be a mild laxative and is soothing to irritated intestines and small children.

The infusion of Elder is used for gargles in cases of sore throat, pharyngitis and mouth infections.

## OTHER USES

Elder is very effective in washing irritated eyes, especially of small children.

If you find yourself in the country and want to keep the insects away from you then rub your face, hands and legs with Elder leaves and you will find out that the insects will never get near you.

## PREPARATION AND DOSAGE

Infusion - soak a handful of Elder flowers in a litre of hot water for ten minutes. You can drink as much as you want and it is recommended for rheumatism, bronchitis and fever.

Tea - put 3-5 grams of dry flowers in a cup of water and leave it for 15 minutes. Drink three cups daily.

Bath - put two handfuls of Elder flowers in a litre of hot water for ten minutes and then pour this infusion in your bath to get relieved from common cold, arthritis or rheumatism.

Liquid extract - use 5 ml for children and 10 ml for adults, twice a day.

Decoction - put one tablespoon of the bark of the herb or the bark of the root in half a cup of water and boil it for two minutes. Leave it to soak for ten minutes and drink of the decoction a mouthful at a time. Do not exceed one cup of the decoction per day.

## SIDE EFFECTS

The fresh herb is quite poisonous, so large quantities should never be used. Its fruit should never be eaten fresh and its juice is extremely dangerous.

If, however, we boil the fruit before we eat it or produce juice out of it, we eliminate the danger. There were reports of dizziness because of frequent use of Elder.

## HISTORY

Elder is one of the most used herbs in traditional medicine. There is evidence that it has been in use from ancient times both for healing purposes as well as for food, especially in dried form. Its leaves were used as an analgesic and for wound healing when made into poultice. American Indians were also familiar with the herb and they were using it for the treatment of cough, wound infections and skin diseases. In the old times, Elder was a symbol of sorrow and grief. This belief may be connected to some stories that say that Judas hanged himself on a big Elder tree or that the Holy Cross was made out of a giant Elder. Even today, there are some superstitions about Elder tree in Europe and is often connected with magic and even haunting.

# Eucalyptus
*Antiseptic, aromatic, antibacterial, stimulant*

**Scientific Name:** Eucalyptus globulus of the Myrtaceae family.

**Parts Used:** leaves.

**USES:** Eucalyptus is used for the treatment of:
- Arthritis
- Asthma
- Cough
- Cold/flu
- Diarrhea
- Herpes
- Cystitis
- Neuralgia
- Fever

Eucalyptus is widely used for cough, asthma, fever, sore throat and neuralgia. Most of the medicines produced from Eucalyptus use the yellowish-green oil derived from its leaves. The lozenges and cough drops made from it are used for colds, coughs, sore throat and lung

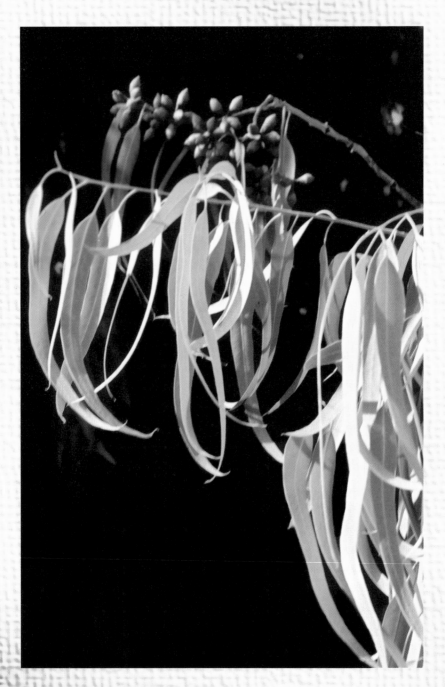

**Eucalyptus**                    112

diseases. Its expectorant properties are useful in bronchitis. The oil is used as a vapor bath for asthma and other respiratory problems, as an antiseptic in the bath and it is also considered that it prevents infections on wounds and burns. A cold extract of the leaves makes a helpful aid for indigestion and fever. Externally, the oil is applied on the body to relieve from rheumatic and neuralgic pains.

## OTHER USES

The oil of Eucalyptus is given to cattle and horses for the treatment of flu and to dogs for bad mood. It is also given to all animals for the treatment of septicaemia (blood poisoning) and skin diseases.

If we place some Eucalyptus leaves in a boll of water and put it to boil, the vapor of the water will spread in the room helping patients with asthma or flu with their respiration. The Eucalyptus vapor kills the bacteria of staphylococcus in the air and protects from the spread of infections.

## PREPARATION AND DOSAGE

Decoction - put 3 leaves of Eucalyptus in a cup of water and put it to boil. When it starts boiling, leave to boil for one minute ad remove it from the fire. Leave the leaves in the water to soak for another ten minutes and then drain the leaves. Drink this decoction 3cups daily.

Infusion - put 25-30 grams of Eucalyptus leaves in a litre of hot water for 10 minutes. Drink one cup, three times daily.

Bath - put 2-3 drops of the Eucalyptus volatile oil in some water.

Breathing - if you are suffering from cold or flu you can ease your breathing using Eucalyptus oil. Put 4 drops of the oil in a bowl of hot water. Add one drop of Thyme and one drop of Green tea and inhale the steam.

## SIDE EFFECTS

Frequent internal use of Eucalyptus volatile oil is not allowed because it affects the kidneys. Caution should be also taken with the quantity of the volatile oil consumed because too much oil may cause serious trouble and even death.

## HISTORY

Eucalyptus is an evergreen tree native to Australia and Tasmania. There are about 300 different species of them and 50 of them grow in the Mediterranean countries.

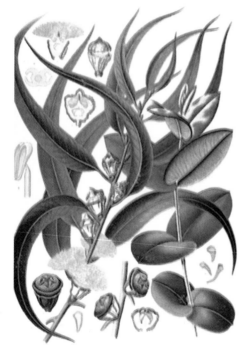

It was widely used in the past for the treatment of intermittent fever. The leaves and their preparations have been successfully used as a tonic and for stimulating the stomach in atonic dyspepsia. Most of Eucalyptus medical uses were revealed to the western world only by the end of the 19th century by the German herbalist Baron Ferdinand von Muller.

# Fennel

*Stomachic, diaphoretic, aromatic, diuretic, perspirative*

**Scientific Name:** Foeniculum vulgare of the Umbelliferae family.

**Parts Used:** seeds, leaves and root.

USES: Fennel is used for the treatment of:
- Weight loss
- Gastric and intestine problems
- Indigestion
- Colic
- Fat accumulation
- Hiccough
- Nausea
- Bad vision

Fennel is used to promote menstrual period in women and also to increase milk production during nursing. As a digestive it accelerates the digestion of fatty food, a property that makes it an excellent remedy for people that try to loose weight. It also soothes colic and stomachic pains while its tea is considered to be helpful in cases of snake and insect bites as well as in food poisoning.

Externally it is used as an eye cleanser and fights gingivitis, swellings and mouth infections.

## OTHER USES

The crashed seeds of Fennel are used as an aromatic spice and gives a wonderful taste to meat, especially fish.

Use a decoction of the seeds or their diluted volatile oil for gargles to get a fresh, aromatised breath.

## PREPARATION AND DOSAGE

Decoction - boil half a teaspoon of crashed seeds in a cup of water for ten to fifteen minutes, keeping it covered throughout the procedure.

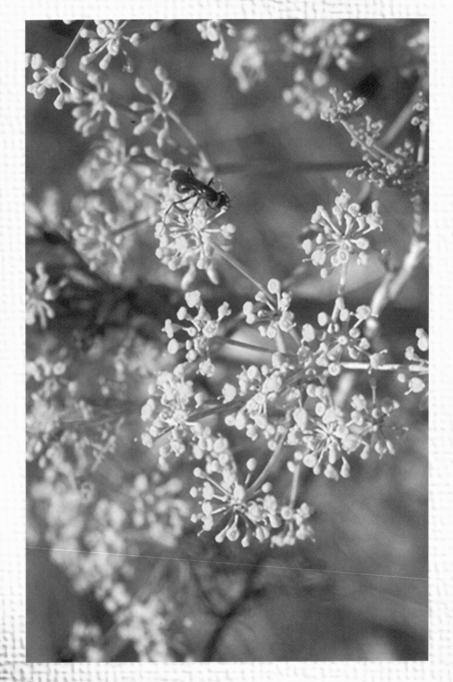

**Fennel**

116

Leave it to cool down, drain the seeds and drink the decoction, three cups daily.

Infusion - very good for indigestion and for losing weight. Put one teaspoon of crashed leaves in one cup of hot water and leave them soak for 15 minutes. Drink a cup after each meal.

Poultice - use the crashed leaves or seeds as a poultice on bruises, wounds and burns.

Oil - Fennel oil is used for massaging swellings and against rheumatism pains. Use 3-5 drops in a tablespoon of honey to help with indigestion, gastric problems and colic.

**SIDE EFFECTS**

No serious side effects resulting from the use of Fennel have been reported. However, it is not recommended in big quantities to pregnant and nursing women as well as to people that have a history of alcoholism, hepatitis or any liver disease. The seeds and leaves of Fennel are extremely safe but its oil may, in some people, cause nausea or vomiting when used internally.

**HISTORY**

It is believed that the Fennel was the source of immortality in the Greek myth of Prometheus. From as early as the $3^{rd}$ century B.C. Fennel was used medicinally and Hippocrates was actually recommending Fennel for child colic. Four hundred years later, Dioscourides suggests that Fennel reduces the appetite and its seeds help nursing mothers to increase their milk production.

Pliny recommends Fennel for 22 different diseases including bad vision or even blindness and jaundice.

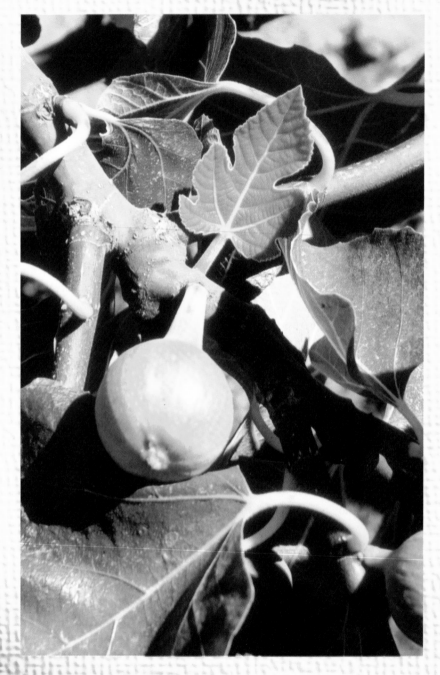

**Figtree**

# Fig tree

*Laxative, emollient, demulcent*

**Scientific Name:** Ficus carica of the Urticaceae family.

**Parts Used:** leaves, fruits and buds.

USES: Fig tree is used for the treatment of:
- Asthma
- Constipation
- Skin rashes
- Smallpox
- Gingivitis, toothache
- Mouth infections
- Pharyngitis
- Abscesses

Figs possess laxative properties and this is why they are used extensively for the production of laxative medicines both for children as well as for adults in syrup form. A milky juice that drips from the Fig's base when cut has miraculous properties on abscesses, skin tumors and other skin problems. Just apply a few drops of this milky juice directly on the area where the problem exists and it will cure the problem in a few days. The action of this juice may cause skin irritations around the area it is applied but they will soon disappear.

A decoction of the dry Figs is very effective for dry, whooping cough and is also used for catarrhal affections of both the throat and the nose. The leaves of Fig tree are used for asthma and when combined with Peppermint they produce an astringent decoction used to stop diarrhea.

## PREPARATION AND DOSAGE

Decoction - boil one big Fig leave in two cups of water until it boils down to half the original quantity of the water. For asthma, drink one cup of this decoction just before bedtime or early in the morning with an empty stomach.

For cough and catarrhal affections, boil three dried Figs in a litre of water until half of the water is left. Drink half a cup every four hours until the cough stops entirely.

Gargles - boil a dried Fig in a cup of milk and use it for gargles to sooth sore throat and mouth infections.

Infusion - put 8 dried figs in a litre of water and leave them to soak for one hour. Drink three cups daily for constipation.

Poultice - boil some fresh Figs for 2-3 minutes and cut them open. The soft inside Figs makes a good poultice for gingivitis, gum abscesses and small skin tumors.


## OTHER USES

Figs are very nutritional and very rich in fibers, natrium, iron and magnesium. In fact, in ancient Greece, Figs were distributed in ratios only to the citizens of Athens and all Fig trees were controlled by the government as they were considered so valuable that their export was strictly forbidden by law.

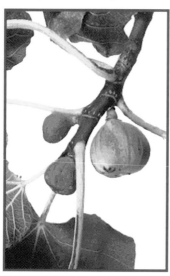

An alcoholic beverage is produced from ripe Figs and in some Mediteranean countries Figs are used in the production of a special wine. And as Pliny reports, Fig wine was produced by ancient Greeks and Romans, centuries ago.

In some Greek islands bread is being produced mixing fresh figs with flour.


## HISTORY

Fig tree grows wild in all the Mediterranean countries but its origin is considered to be the Middle East and specifically Persia, Syria and Asia Minor. The Greeks imported it from Caria, Asia Minor, a place where Fig tree has derived its scientific name from (Ficus carica) and it was under the Greek cultivation that it became known to the rest of Europe. It was so esteemed in Greece for its nutritional value that athletes were fed entirely on Figs. Fig tree was dedicated to Bacchus and was used during the religious ceremonies that were held in his favor. Figs were also known to Romans from the very early days and it is mentioned in the Latin mythology. In early Roman times, it was considered to be a sacred tree because Remus and Romulus were fed by a wolf under a Fig tree.

Fig tree was also mentioned by Homer, Ovid, Pliny, Varro, Dioscourides and Theophrastus who described both its nutritional and medicinal uses in the past.

# Flax
*Antiseptic, emollient, pectoral, demulcent*

**Scientific Name:** Linum usitatissimum of the Linaceae family.

**Parts Used:** seeds.

USES: Flax is used for the treatment of:
- Abscesses
- Jaundice
- Urinary organs irritation
- Skin infections
- Acme

Its poultice is used externally for abscesses, skin infections, acme and burns soothing the pain and promoting suppuration. Internally, the seeds are valuable for jaundice, irritation of the urinary system and inflammations. It is also used for common colds, coughs, pneumonia and pains due to rheumatism while its emollient properties make the herb useful in constipation.

## PREPARATION AND DOSAGE

Infusion - put three tablespoons of Flaxseeds in a litre of water and leave them soak for one whole night. Add some honey and maybe some lemon juice to sweeten it and drink 3 cups per day.

Decoction - boil one tablespoon of Flaxseeds in a cup of water until it boils down to half its original volume. Leave it to cool down and drink it.

Oil - Linseed oil is very useful externally but can also be used internally as a laxative and against all kinds of inflammations as well as for Jaundice.

Poultice - boil the Flaxseeds until they become soft and sticky when touched. Before they cool down, place them in a dry cloth and apply them on the place we want.

## OTHER USES

Linseed oil is used in paint manufacturing as well as for the production of printing inks. The residue of the seeds (from where the oil has been extracted) offer a nutritional food for cattle, sheep and even birds.

The oil is also used as a veterinary medicine for cattle and sheep.

## HISTORY

There is proven evidence that Flax was used in the ancient times for cloth making. Flax woven garments were found in ancient Egyptian tombs while linen cloths are mentioned in the Bible, both the Old and the New Testament. It is mentioned that the clothing of Jesus Christ in his tomb was made out of Flax.

# Garlic

*One of the most important herbs, recommended for*
*many diseases especially of the circulatory system*

**Scientific Name:** Allium
sativum of the Liliaceae family.

**Parts Used:** bulb.

USES: Garlic is used for the
treatment of:
- Arteriosclerosis
- Hypertension
- High cholesterol
- High triglycerides
- Congestive heart failure
- Neuralgias
- Infections
- Blood coagulation

Garlic is probably the most researched herb. There are hundreds of
books written about it and its medicinal properties. Since the ancient
times, we have evidence of the use of Garlic for the treatment of a big
number of diseases. It is mentioned in the Bible as well as in the Talmud
and other ancient scripts and is also found in the writings of Hippocrates,
Dioscourides, Pliny and almost every single famous physician or
herbalist. In China its use has been confirmed to have started by 510 B.C.
while the first scientific proof came from Louis Pasteur in 1858 when he
confirmed Garlic's antibacterial action experimenting in his lab.

Garlic has some unmatched properties that no other herb has. It
reduces cholesterol and the levels of triglyceride in the blood; expands
the blood arteries, reducing in this way the pressure in hypertensive
people (people with high blood pressure); it acts as a natural anti-
coagulant inhibiting the platelet stickiness on artery walls; it reduces the
risk of certain cancers inhibiting the formation of carcinogenic
compounds; long term use of Garlic has been proven to fight
arteriosclerosis. These properties do not mean of course that Garlic may
replace some stronger chemical medicines but population studies have

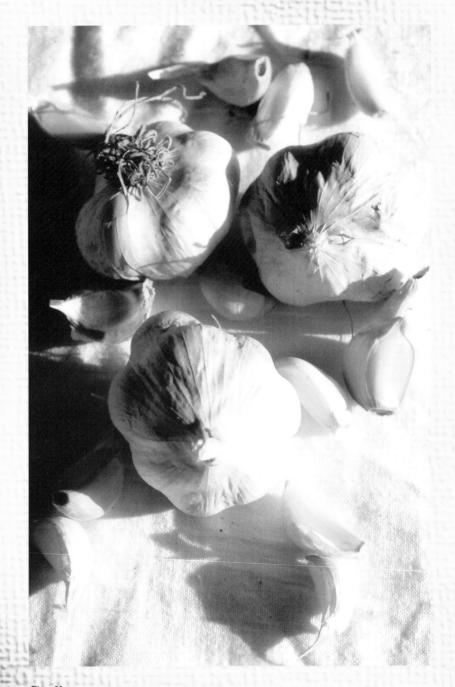

**Garlic** 124

proved that long term use of Garlic is preventive against a variety of serious diseases. For years it has been used preventively for reducing the risk of cardiovascular diseases and it is also used to fight bacteria and parasites of the intestine. Garlic is definitely an excellent herb and a lot have been written about it but we should not rely on just its use in serious diseases. We should always consult our doctor if we are under treatment for diseases of the cardiovascular system before using Garlic or any of its preparations because some medicines have been found to interact with it.

## A HOPE AGAINST CANCER

Most of the scientific research performed during the last two decades focused on Garlic's activity against cancer. Statistical studies has shown that communities that eat Garlic on a regular basis report much less cases of a variety of cancers like that of the esophagus, the stomach and the intestines. This has been associated with Garlic's ability to induce the formation of carcinogenic compounds, an ability that has not yet been explained. Lab experiments on animals have also proved that Garlic prevents or even stops carcinogenesis in cancers of the skin and the breast.

## OTHER USES

Everyone knows of course of the use of Garlic in the kitchen. Another use of Garlic is mixing it with animal food, raw and finely cut, as a remedy for preventing various intestine and stomachic diseases.

An alcoholic preparation made out of 4 bulbs of Garlic in a litre of plain spirit produces a good stimulant for falling hair and even baldness.

## PREPARATION AND DOSAGE

There is no better way to take Garlic other than the fresh, natural bulb. Unfortunately, despite the so many benefits of fresh Garlic, its smell is very unpleasant and this is the main reason why most people avoid it, especially in the Western countries. Nevertheless, there are dozens of preparations of Garlic in the market (pills, capsules, syrups, etc) that contain almost all the valuable ingredients of Garlic (not all) but do not have the unpleasant smell of the fresh herb.

A homemade syrup for asthma and other lung diseases can be easily prepared using fresh bulbs. Clean the skin of 100 grams of Garlic bulbs and boil them in half a litre of water until the bulbs become soft. Add vinegar at the same quantity as the remaining water and boil the mixture for another 10 minutes. Remove the bulbs, add sugar and continue boiling the mixture until it becomes a smooth syrup. Then put the bulbs in a small pot and pour the syrup on top of them. Take one tablespoon a day containing one bulb per spoon.

## SIDE EFFECTS

The biggest problem with Garlic is its strong unpleasant smell. A quick solution is to chew a couple of Basil leaves right after eating Garlic but this will only last for half an hour. Garlic smell lasts until its complete digestion and sometimes it is even mixed with the sweat of the person eating it so there is actually no easy way to avoid Garlic smell if we want to eat it fresh. Even some preparations that do not really smell Garlic may make a person smell garlic through his or her perspiration.

Persons with heart problems, high pressure or other serious diseases should consult their doctor if they want to use Garlic on regular basis especially patients that take anti-coagulant medications with which Garlic may interact.

People with weak stomach may experience heartburn or flatulence after taking fresh Garlic or even some of its preparations.

## HISTORY

According to Theophrastus, ancient Greeks used to put fresh Garlic on stone piles at crossroads for Hecate to eat. Pliny says that Garlic and Onion were offered to their gods when taking oaths.

126

Hippocrates recommended Garlic for a lot of diseases and ancient Greeks used to eat it on a daily basis although Horace mentions that the smell of Garlic was actually detested by the noble class. Hundreds of writers from the days of the Old Testament until today have written about Garlic and lots of myths and superstitions were created around this precious herb.

# Gentian

*An excellent appetizer, tonic, blood cleanser*
*and curative to peptic problems.*

**Scientific Name:** Gentian lutea of the Gentianaceae family.

**Parts Used:** Root.

**Uses:** Gentian is used for the treatment of:
- Anorexia
- Malfunctions of the peptic system
- Dyspepsia (indigestion)
- Hysteria
- Rabbies

Gentian is considered to be one of the most useful bitter tonic herbs. It is used as an appetizer in general and it is thought to be therapeutic in cases of anorexia. It is used in cases of exhaustion from chronic diseases and in cases of weakness of the digestive organs, strengthening the human organism by purifying the blood. This property of the herb helps human organs such as the liver, the heart and the spleen to function better. It has relieving properties in cases of stomach and intenstine complaints and acts instantly against indigestion. Gentian will also help women that suffer form hysteria and nervousness and the powder of its dry roots has

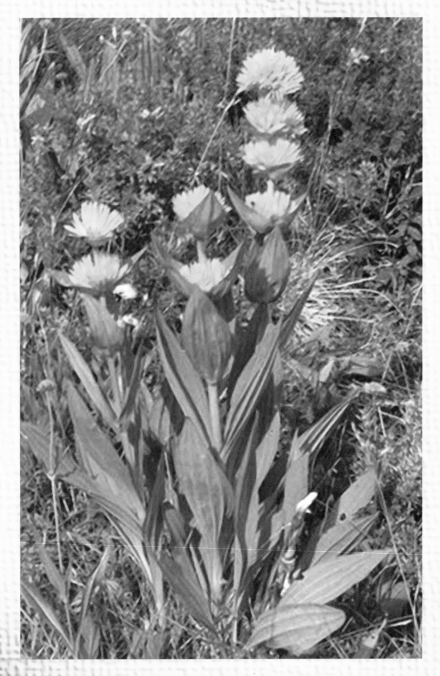

**Gentian**                    128

been used for centuries on the bites from rage dogs and venomous beasts, both on humans and animals.

## PREPARATION AND DOSAGE

Tincture - put one teaspoon of dried, finely cut (or powdered) Gentian root in one litre of water and leave it through the night. In the morning we can drain the water and drink one cup of it at least 15 minutes before meals.

Wine - steep two tablespoons of Gentian in one litre of wine and leave it for about a week. Drinking of that wine will refresh weak and weary people.

## OTHER USES

In a lot of European countries and especially Germany, Gentian root is used for the production of alcoholic beverages, which are usually drunk as aperitif before dinner.

## SIDE EFFECTS

Gentian should not be used by people with stomach ulcers, gastritis or heartburn and also by hypertensive people.

## HISTORY

According to Pliny and Dioscourides, Gentian derived its name from an ancient Greek King, the King of Illyria (180-167 B.C.) named Gentius. According to the two botanologists, Gentius was the first to discover the curative properties of the herb and so it was named after him. Gentians are actually a big group of plants, numbering about 180 species which are found around the world in different forms and colours. In Europe, the blue Gentian is the most abundant, with yellow and white being rarer. In South America on the contrary, we will find red Gentian in abundance. The Gentian referred in this book is the yellow Gentian.

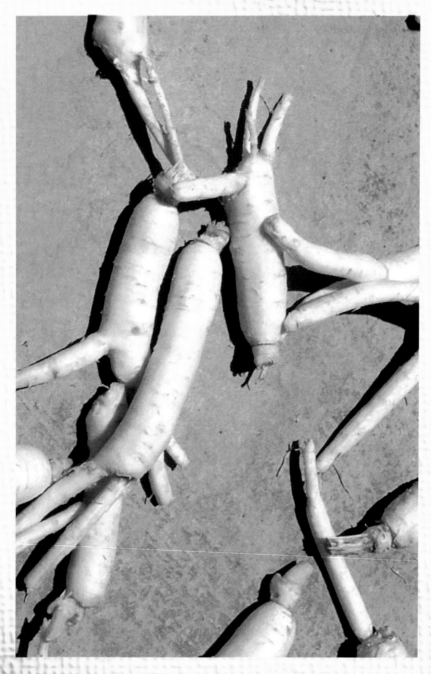

**Ginseng (asian)** 130

# Ginseng (Asian)

*Known as the king of all herbs, it is an excellent tonic, aphrodisiac and fights stress.*

**Scientific Name:** Panax ginseng of the Araliaceae family.

**Parts Used:** Root.

**Uses:** Ginseng is used for the treatment of:
- Stress
- Arteriosclerosis
- Amnesia
- Anorexia
- Alzheimers disease
- Mental and nervous exhaustion
- Diabetes
- Fibromyalgia
- Depression
- Male impotense
- Chemotherapy (support during its course)
- Menstruation complaints

Ginseng is an excellent herb for mental, nervous and general exhaustion. The Chinese respected and loved Ginseng almost like a God and they considered the herb panacea to all human diseases for a few millenniums now. There are a lot of myths that refer to Ginseng as a gift from God or as the cure of all diseases, mental and physical, mostly due to its roots that resemble very much the human body.

USES: Ginseng has been used as a tonic in ancient China and other Asian countries and is now being used as such all over the world. It is known to strengthen the nervous system and has the ability to clear the toxins from the human body and increase the oxygen circulation in the blood.

Stress - It is believed that Ginseng fights stress and some mood disorders.

Menstruation - women are using Ginseng to normalise their menstrual period and other "female" problems even easing childbirth.

Anorexia / Digestion - It helps against anorexia and digestion disorders, since it is a mild stimulant to the nervous system and to various glands.

Exhaustion - One of the most valuable properties of Ginseng is its tonic power. As mentioned above it stimulates the central nervous system and increases mental and biological stamina and endurance.

Diabetes - It is recommended to diabetics for stabilising their metabolism and normalising blood sugar levels.

Flu - Ginseng is used preventively against common cold and flu or during the illness to strengthen the human body fight the illness.

## PREPARATION AND DOSAGE

The active ingredients of Ginseng are found in its roots. These roots can be mixed with wine to form a tonic beverage or can be finely cut or powdered (after they are dried) to be consumed as they are, either by chewing the root or by placing the powder under the tongue.

Of course today Ginseng is widely spread and you will be able to find a Ginseng product in almost any pharmacy. Standardised Ginseng extracts are considered to be the most reliable. The most effective forms are the ones standardised to 4-7% of ginsenosides. More concentrated extracts not only they are not better but they are less effective due to the reduction of panaxan levels. The daily dosage of standardised extracts varies from 100 to 200 mg.

The dosage for non standardised extracts is relatively higher, about 1-2 grams per day in tablet form or 2-3ml daily in tincture form of the fresh herb. The dried root of the herb can also be used for tea if you prefer it. In general Ginseng is taken for 2-3 weeks continuously a break of 1-2 weeks follows and then start taking it again.

## SIDE EFFECTS

It is advised not to take Ginseng in combination with other stimulants, even coffee, in large quantities or to be given to people being treated with hormonic medication or antiphychotic drugs. The best thing to do before you start taking Ginseng in combination with any other medications is to consult your doctor. Ginseng is also not allowed to people with fever or they are neurotic or hysteric. If after taking Ginseng for a few days you develop insomnia, nervousness, diarrhea or skin rashes, it is better to stop taking it for a while to check if the problem is due to the herb.

## HISTORY

Ginseng is probably the most widely known herb in the world today but it was only recently imported in the Western countries compared to China where its curative and tonic properties have been known for 5000 to 7000 years. Its scientific name Panax is derived from the Greek word Panakia, a synthetic word of the words Pan Aksos that have the meaning of cure all.

On the other hand, the word Ginseng is said to have another two meanings: "the root of life" and "the wonder of the world".

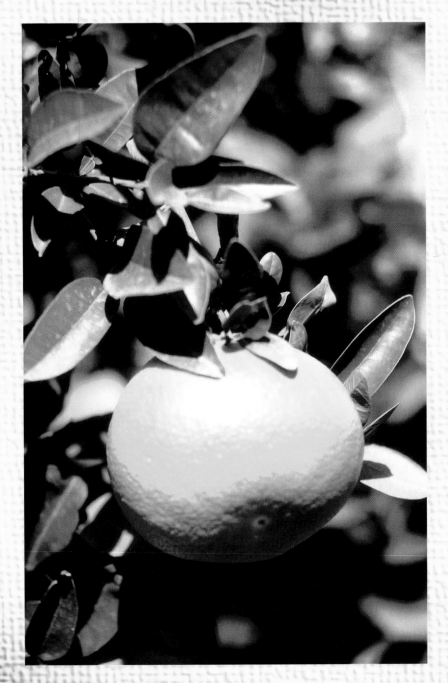

**Grapefruit** 134

# Grapefruit

*Digestive, stomachic, antiseptic, tonic, diuretic*

**Scientific Name:** Citrus paradisi of the Rutaceae family.

**Parts Used:** fruits.

**USES**: Grapefruit is used for the treatment of:
- Digestion
- Liver
- High cholesterol
- Cancer
- Excess fat

Grapefruit is an excellent supplement to be included in diets of people trying to lose weight. Its ingredients help in reducing your appetite and are very low in calories (100 grams of Grapefruit contain only 30-33 calories). There is a lot of research being performed to find out the effects of Grapefruit on cancer. A study in Montreal in 1997 showed that mice drinking Grapefruit juice instead of water had 50% less tumors than mice in the same study drinking pure water. Pink and red Grapefruit reduce the risk of developing prostate cancer.

Grapefruit has been found to have a positive effect on the liver while another clinical study on animals showed that Grapefruit juice reduced Cholesterol levels by 32%.

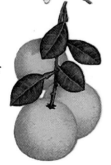

## OTHER USES

People suffering from arthritis and other inflammatory diseases may reduce the frequency and the strength of their disease's symptoms by drinking Grapefruit juice on a daily basis.

## SIDE EFFECTS

People allergic to Citrus fruit will most probably react to Grapefruit too. This reaction might be caused by the fruit itself or the oil of its skin.

Also, the juice of the fruit inhibits a special enzyme in the intestines that is responsible for metabolising some chemical medicines. Therefore certain medicines should not be combined with Grapefruit (see medicine interactions at the end of this book) so consult your doctor if you are under medical treatment.

# Green tea
*Antioxidant, tonic, astringent, fights cancer*

**Scientific Name:** Camelia sinensis of the Camelliaceae family.

**Parts Used:** the dried leaves.

**USES:** Green tea is used for the treatment of:
- Infections
- Gingivitis
- Immune function
- Cancer
- High cholesterol
- Hypertension
- High triglycerides

It helps in the prevention of flu, hypertension and infections and boosts the immune system of the organism protecting the body from the atmospheric pollution. It is used to reduce cholesterol and triglyceride levels in the blood and is recommended for headaches and pains on any part of the body. In addition, it reduces high blood pressure, fights diarrhea, revives the function of most body organs and helps in teeth hygiene.

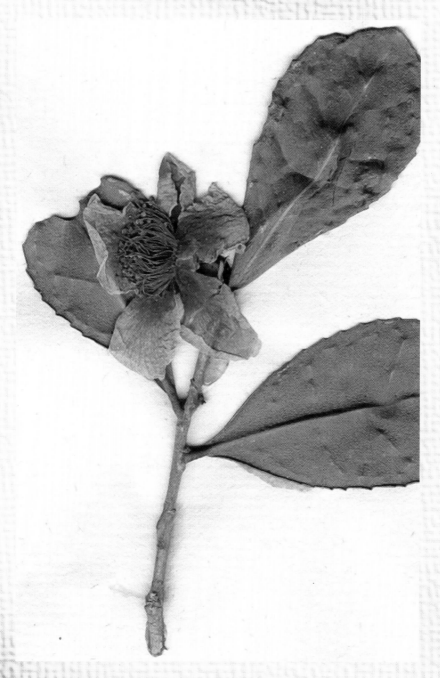

137 **Green tea**

Most of the scientific research on Green tea is focused in the effect of the herb in fighting or preventing cancer. A series of studies on animals has shown that the polyphenols contained in Green tea offer significant protection against cancer. Green tea is at least ten times more protective against cancer than black tea. In fact, Black tea increases the risk of certain cancers like the cancer of the gallbladder, the endometrium and the rectum. Both Green tea and Black tea are derived from the same plant but using different methods of preparation. Green tea is not fermented, unlike the Black tea, so the active ingredients and especially the polyphenols remain unaltered in the herb.

Green tea also affects positively the function of the liver, the womb, the breast, the peptic system and the lungs.

## OTHER USES

Certain research has shown that a cup of Green tea suppresses the complications of anaemia.

## PREPARATION AND DOSAGE

Infusion - soak one teaspoon of Green tea leaves in a cup of boiling water and leave it for three minutes. Drink as much of it as you want, but do not overdo it.

## SIDE EFFECTS

Green tea is very safe to use. The most known side effects (related to over consumption) are insomnia, excitement and other symptoms that are caused from the caffeine that it contains.

Large quantities may also provoke indigestion and sudden weakness.

## HISTORY

First of all we have to make it clear that Green tea is a specific tea and has nothing to do with mountain tea. It is also known as Chinese or Ceylon tea.

It is not yet known exactly when and where the use of Green tea started. According to a Chinese myth, its use was accidentally discovered by an emperor, 4000 years ago. The first written evidence, is in the Chinese ancient dictionary that places the use of Green tea back to 350 B.C. Since then, traditional Chinese medicine recommends it for headaches, indigestion, depression, pain, toxicity, energy and generally for life longevity. It became known to Europe only in the seventeenth century when it was brought by Dutch and Portuguese settlers. Modern medicine has confirmed a lot of the recommendations of Chinese traditional medicine.

# Hawthorn
*Heart tonic, sedative, antispasmodic, vasodilator*

**Scientific Name:** Crataegus oxyacantha of the Rosaceae family.

**Parts Used:** flowers, leaves and fruit.

**USES:** Hawthorn is used for the treatment of:
- Angina pectoris
- Arteriosclerosis
- Congestive heart failure
- Hypertension
- Insomnia

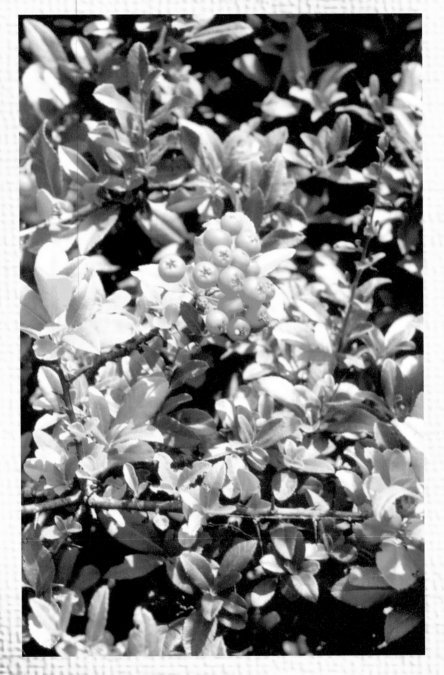

**Hawthorn** 140

Heart - Hawthorn is excellent for treating both high and low blood pressure by strengthening the heart function. It strengthens the heart muscles increasing in this way the pumping power of this vital organ. It may open up the coronary arteries, supplying more blood to the heart, and it seems to reduce the amount of cholesterol deposited on the walls of the arteries. There are cases reported where Hawthorn has helped in eliminating arrhythmias (problems of the heart related to its rhythm). Hawthorn is considered one of the most valuable herbs for treating heart problems.

Although there are a lot of preparations of Hawthorn being sold at the pharmacies, any heart disease is a serious condition and Hawthorn does not take action right away, so always consult your doctor for your condition and advice. It can however be taken as a prevenive measure to prevent angina pectoris, arteriosclerosis, blood globing and high blood pressure.

Insomnia - Hawthorn is also a mild sedative and might be very helpful in cases of anxiousness, insomnia and nervous breakdowns.

**PREPARATION AND DOSAGE**

Decoction - boil one or two teaspoons of Hawthorn flowers in one litre of water for 5 minutes. You can drink it as a sedative, 2-3 times daily.

Infusion - put two teaspoons of Hawthorn leaves cut into small pieces or Hawthorn berries in a cup of boiling water for 20 minutes. Drain it and drink two cups of it per day.

Tincture - 4 to 5 ml, three times daily.

Capsules/tablets - the dose is between 80-300 mg of standardised extract but if taken in its natural form take 4-5 grams of the herb per day.

## SIDE EFFECTS

Although there are no side effects reported for Hawthorn, large quantities and continuous use may cause sedation and blood pressure reduction. In some cases this may be good but not always, so consult your doctor if you suffer from any disease of the circulatory system or any heart problems.

## HISTORY

The scientific name of Hawthorn, Crataegus Oxyacantha is derived from the Greek "Krateos" meaning strong (the hard wood of Hawthorn), "oxy" meaning sharp and "acantha" meaning thorn. The English name Hawthorn is derived from the use of it like a hedge to divide the fields between them. "Haw" is actually an old English word for hedge. Its use though was not limited in hedge making but was definitely used as a medicine as well. From the time of the famous Greek herbalist Dioscourides, the first century B.C., Hawthorn has been used to treat diseases of the circulatory system and the heart but it was only during the last two centuries that the use of the herb expanded to the whole world. In fact, Hawthorn preparations are prescribed to heart patients even today, especially in Germany and central Europe.

# Ivy

*Antispasmodic, anti-neuralgic, anticoagulant*

**Scientific Name:** Hedera helix of the Araliaceae family.

**Parts Used:** the whole plant (flowering).

**USES:** Ivy is used for the treatment of:
- Dysentery
- Pains
- Burns
- Throat diseases
- Gall bladder stones

It is used internally for cocitis, chronic bronchitis and laryngitis and also for the dilution of gallstones. Due to its anti-neuralgic and anticoagulant properties it is a very good remedy for arthritis, neuralgias, blood glotting, varicose veins, wound healing, burns ($1^{st}$ and $2^{nd}$ degree) and phlebitis. It is also used externally for pain relief, burns, wounds, otitis and toothache.

## PREPARATION AND DOSAGE

Decoction for internal use - put 3 tablespoons of finely cut, fresh Ivy leaves in a litre of water and heat it for ten minutes. Drain it and drink 3 cups per day.

Decoction for external use - put one handful of dry Ivy leaves in a litre of water and heat them for ten minutes. Use it for baths or add plenty of salt to use it for gargles.

Poultice - apply the fresh leaves on the wound or the burn and replace them when they start drying. They absorb the pus and help the wound to heal.

Wine - a decoction of the flowers in wine restrains dysentery.

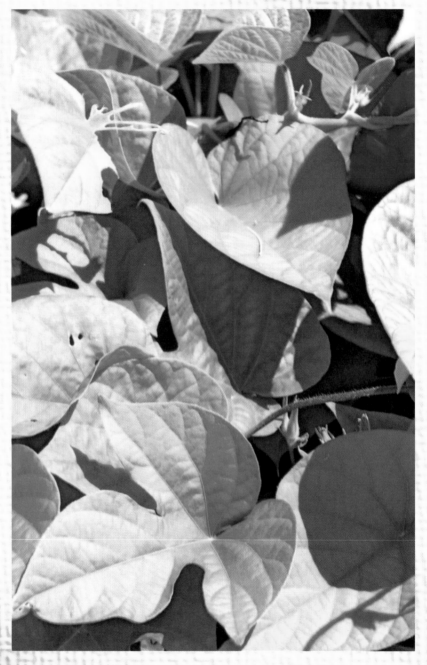

**Ivy**

144

## SIDE EFFECTS

If we use Ivy internally in large quantities, it may cause poisoning. Poisoning from Ivy provokes vomiting, diarrhea and acute irritation of the stomach and the intestines. We should also avoid the use of black Ivy (the bushy one that does not climb) which is very toxic and may cause poisoning if used the same way common Ivy is used.

## HISTORY

Ivy was the main plant during the Dionysos feasts. The ancient Greeks used to make wreaths out of it during these feasts, they would chew its leaves and drink its decoction in combination with wine, making them drunk with hallucinations that would always result to an orgy. The Greek priests presented a wreath of Ivy to newly married couples as it was regarded to be a symbol of fidelity. The custom of decorating houses and churches with Ivy during Christmas was forbidden by one of the early Councils of the Church because of its pagan association.

# Knotgrass
*Astringent, diuretic, wound healing*

**Scientific Name:** Polygonum vulgare of the Polygonaceae family.

**Parts Used:** the whole flowering plant.

USES: Knotgrass is used for the treatment of:
- Diarrhea
- Bleeding
- Colic
- Rheumatic pains

145

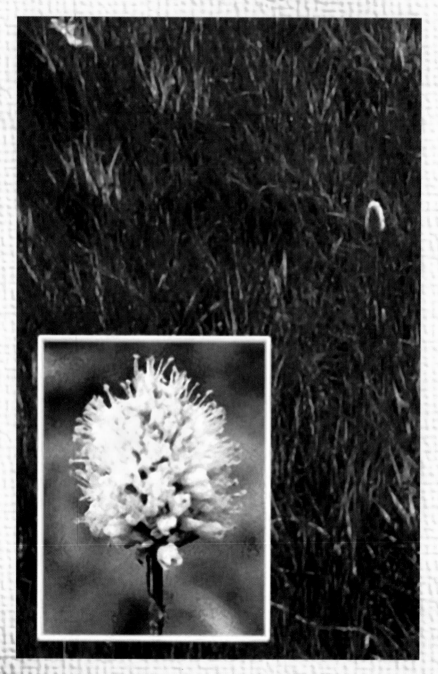

**Knotgrass**

146

The astringent properties of Knotgrass make its infusion useful for diarrhea, hemorrhoids and rheumatic pains. It is also used as a diuretic especially in cases of painful urination or uraemia.

It is used internally to stop nose bleeding and generally all kinds of bleeding and its decoction kills worms and parasites of the intestines.

### PREPARATION AND DOSAGE

Infusion - put two teaspoons of the herb in a cup of hot water for 10 minutes and drain it. Drink one to three cups daily.

Decoction - boil two teaspoons of the herb in a cup of water for ten minutes. Cover it and let it cool down and then drain it. Drink three cups daily. You can also use the decoction externally in compresses.

Poultice - mash the herb into pulp and use it on wounds or hemorrhoids.

# Laurel (Bay)
*Antiseptic, sedative, spasmolytic*

**Scientific Name:** Laurus nobilis of the Lauraceae family.

**Parts Used:** leaves and fruit.

**USES:** Laurel is used for the treatment of:
- Arthritis
- Fever
- Rheumatism
- Stomach ache
- Falling hair

Laurel is considered to be stomach tonic and there are quite a few

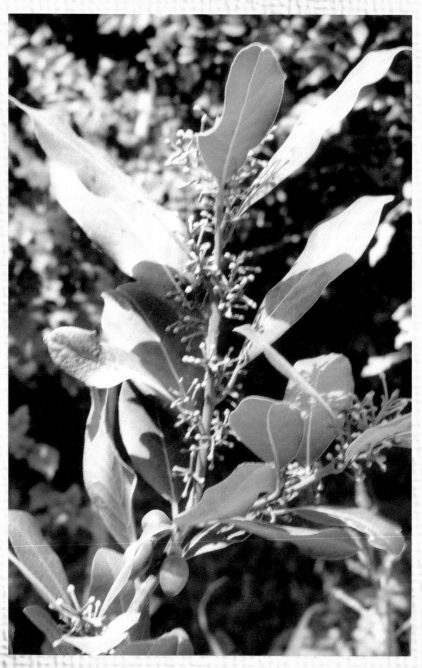

**Laurel (Bay)** 148

preparations prepared for this purpose.

Laurel leaves are also tonic and they are used for indigestion, rheumatism, arthritis and fever. In large quantities they are used to provoke vomiting (emetic) while the dry powder of the leaves stops nose bleeding if used locally.

Its essential oil has similar properties and is very effective for flatulence, arthritis and rheumatism.

Laurel oil inhibits falling hair while it is often used to strengthen the hair and resumes the dark color of black hair. It is also used on bruises.

## OTHER USES

The essential oil of Laurel is used in soap manufacturing and food processing industry.

The leaves are widely used in cooking as a spice.

## PREPARATION AND DOSAGE

Decoction - put three Laurel leaves in a cup of water for three minutes. If one cup is drunk after dinner it acts as a digestive aid and as a mild sedative that promotes sleep.

Compresses - put ten dry Laurel leaves in one cup of hot water and cover the cup for about ten minutes. Drain the leaves and use the water for compresses that can be used for fever, neuralgia or even igmoritis.

## SIDE EFFECTS

Laurel oil should never be used undiluted directly on the skin because it may cause rashes or even burns. Women should also be careful in using Laurel berries (the fruit) because they are often used to discontinue pregnancy.

Internally, Laurel oil may cause vomiting or nausea so drink it with caution and always diluted.


## HISTORY

The word Laurel is connected with heroism and heroic actions, and is sometimes used metaphorically in this sense. This may have been derived from an ancient Greek tradition where all the warriors returning from a victory were crowned by a Laurel wreath. This tradition was later expanded to include athletes, poets and philosophers and was transferred to the Romans. In the ancient times, Laurel leaves symbolised victory, wisdom and poetry. Even today, Laurel leaves symbolise victory and fame.

According to the Greek mythology, Daphne (the Greek name for Laurel) was an extremely beautiful girl, daughter of Mother Earth, that was being hunted by the God Apollo. When he finally managed to reach her, she called for help to her mother and Mother Earth took her away and placing a Laurel tree in her place. This is why Laurel was very important in Apollo worship and generally in the everyday life of ancient Greeks.

At the oracle of Apollo in Delphi, the priestess Pythia used to chew Laurel leaves before she was ready to foretell the future.

150

# Lavender

*Analgesic, sedative, antiseptic,*
*antibacterial, heart tonic*

**Scientific Name:** Lavandula officinalis of the Labiatae family.

**Parts Used:** leaves and flowers.

**USES**: Lavender is used for the treatment of:
- Migraine/headache
- Nervous disorders
- Insomnia
- Poisoning
- Wounds, eczema, burns skin infections

Lavender is a beautiful herb used internally in decoction form to relieve from migraine, headaches (especially those resulting from stress), dizziness, fainting and insomnia. It possesses the property to boost the nervous system while at the same time it is calming in cases of nervous breakdown, depression and anxiety.

It is antispasmodic to diseases of the respiratory system like asthma, bronchitis, tuberculosis and flu. Lavender is also known for its ability to reduce high blood pressure in hypertensive people and it is often used as tonic for the heart, regulating the circulatory system.

It is a strong antiseptic and antibacterial and as such is used externally to accelerate wound healing and internally for cystitis. Its tonic action helps in exhaustion and promotes natural sleep. Finally it has been used as an antidote to poisoning.

## PREPARATION AND DOSAGE

Decoction - boil one tablespoon of Lavender flowers in a cup of water for five minutes and leave them to soak in the water for another ten

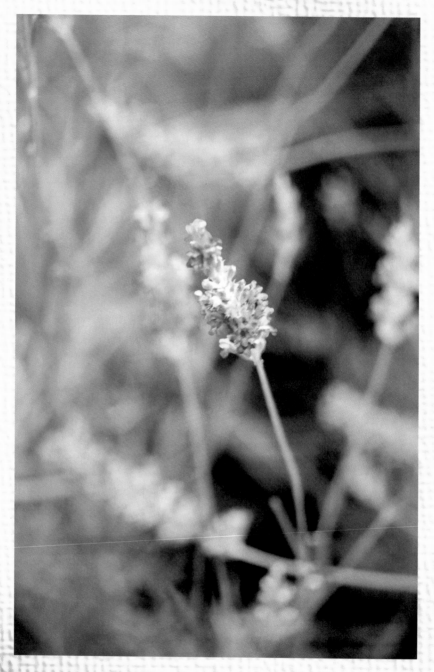

**Lavender**

minutes covering the pot with a cloth. Drink three to four cups daily.

Infusion - put a handful of the flowers in a litre of hot water and leave them soaking for 15 minutes. Drain the flowers and drink three cups daily.

External use - boil one handful of Lavender flowers in a litre of water for ten minutes. Use the decoction on a cloth for applying it on the wounds, for massage and for gargles.

## SIDE EFFECTS

The herb should be avoided in large quantities. People suffering from stomach problems should not use Lavender because it irritates the stomach. Lavender volatile oil should only be used externally because its internal use in large quantities is narcotic and may cause problems that can be even fatal. The frequent use of Lavender decoction or infusion may cause colic.

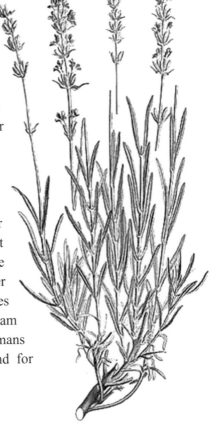

## HISTORY

The healing properties of Lavender place the herb in the group of the most widely used herbs in the world. There is actually a big demand for Lavender and France alone produces 1,500 tones of Lavender volatile oil with steam distillation per year. The ancient Romans used to bath in Lavender water and for scenting their clothes.

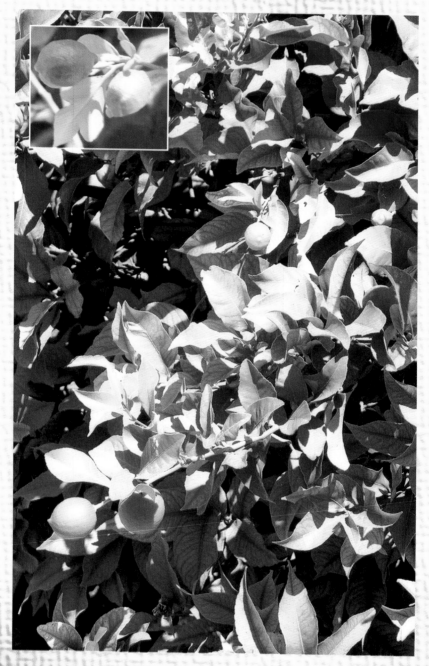

**Lemon**

# Lemon
*Antiscorbutic, antiseptic, astringent,*
*stimulant, carminative, diuretic*

**Scientific Name:** Citrus limonum of the Rutaceae family.

**Parts Used:** flowers, leaves, fruit, skin and seeds.

**USES:** Lemon is used for the treatment of:
- Arthritis
- Sore throat
- Indigestion
- Fever
- Rheumatism
- Freckles
- Abnormal menstrual period
- Thrombosis
- Cough
- Dundruff

Lemon is probably the best antiscorbutic. English ships are required by law to carry enough lemon juice so that each seaman takes about 30 grams per day if the ship travels continuously for more than ten days. It soothes sore throat with gargles and its juice is used for the treatment of rheumatism and arthritis. The decoction is often used to reduce the body temperature in fevers and even typhoid.

### OTHER USES
Lemon rind and its juice are used as an aromatic in medicines, sweets and beverages.

Lemon is of course rich in vitamin C and is often used as a preventive measure to winter colds.

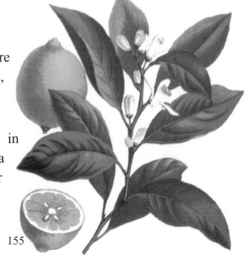

155

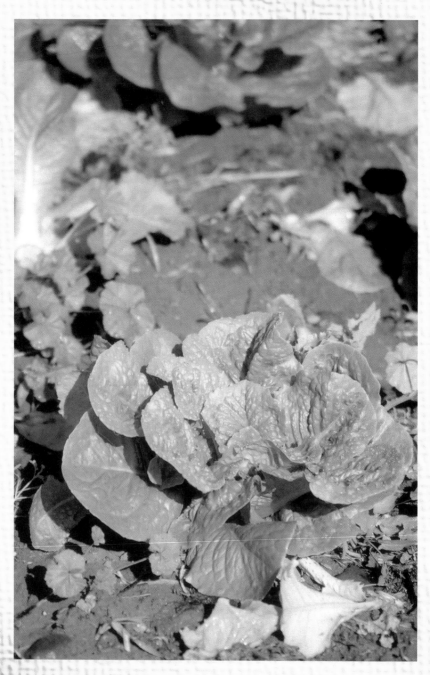

**Lettuce (wild)** 156

# Lettuce (wild)

### Sedative, diuretic, antispasmodic, anodyne, fights insomnia

**Scientific Name:** Lactusa virosa of the Compositae family.

**Parts Used:** leaves and its white juice.

USES: Lettuce is used for the treatment of:
- Insomnia
- Asthma
- Dropsy
- Kidney stones
- Jaundice
- Cough

Cutting the fresh lettuce from its base, it will drip a white milky juice that has similar properties to opium but without the stomach and enteric upsets that the latter causes. This juice can be used, in the right quantities, as a sleeping aid or even as a narcotic. The leaves of Lettuce have similar properties but in a smaller degree, that is why a Lettuce salad at night is very good for people with insomnia. A decoction using dry leaves of Lettuce is a strong diuretic, helps in cases of kidney stones, soothes colic pains and dry cough and is also antispasmodic and helps patients with asthma. It also has sedative properties with overactive children and in cases of overstrain and excitement. Finally, Lettuce may soothe muscle stiffness or pain that accompanies rheumatism.

## OTHER USES

The fresh vegetable is of course used for the preparation of nice salads. Its white juice is also used as a narcotic on small animals and sometimes it is so strong that it causes death.

## PREPARATION AND DOSAGE

Decoction - boil two teaspoons of dry Lettuce leaves in a cup of water for 5 minutes and leave them to soak for another ten minutes. Drink it while hot.

Juice - the milky juice that drips from Lettuce right after it has been cut. Cut the Lettuce from its base with a sharp knife and let it "sit" on an empty glass so that the juice drips into the glass. This juice can be used at once or we can leave it to dry for later use.

## SIDE EFFECTS

As it has been already mentioned, Lettuce juice is a strong narcotic, so its use is not recommended in large doses.

## HISTORY

Wild Lettuce usually grows near the banks of rivers and the lakes. Its cultivation originated from Europe, from where it spread to the USA and eventually to the rest of the world. In the old times, Lettuce was mostly used because of its refreshing properties rather than its curative, with the exception of ancient Rome where Lettuce was highly esteemed among medicinal herbs. It is even reported by historians that the emperor Augustus built a big temple dedicated to Lettuce because it saved him from a serious disease.

# Licorice

*Anti-inflammatory, antispasmodic, tonic, sedative, emetic, laxative, anti-hepatotoxic*

**Scientific Name:** Glycyrrhiza glabra of the Leguminosae family.

**Parts Used:** Root.

**USES:** Licorice is used for the treatment of:
- Asthma
- Cough
- Gastric ulcers
- Flu and cold
- Fatigue

Liver - Licorice is widely used, especially in Japan, for its antioxidant properties on the liver and has been found to be very helpful for the treatment of chronic hepatitis and liver cirrhosis. A lot of studies in Europe and some Asian countries focused on Glycyrrhizin (an active ingredient of Licorice that is 50-60 times sweeter than white sugar). This substance enhances the antibody production of the organism and has been found to repair the liver cells that have been injured by carbon tetrachloride, benzene hexachloride and PCB. It also inhibits the growth of several DNA and RNA viruses like the one in herpes. Other medicinal uses of Licorice include gastritis, peptic ulcers and bronchitis.

**OTHER USES**

Sugar produced from Licorice can be consumed safely by diabetics. The root is also used as a sweetener and aromatic in medicine, confectionery, alcoholic beverages,

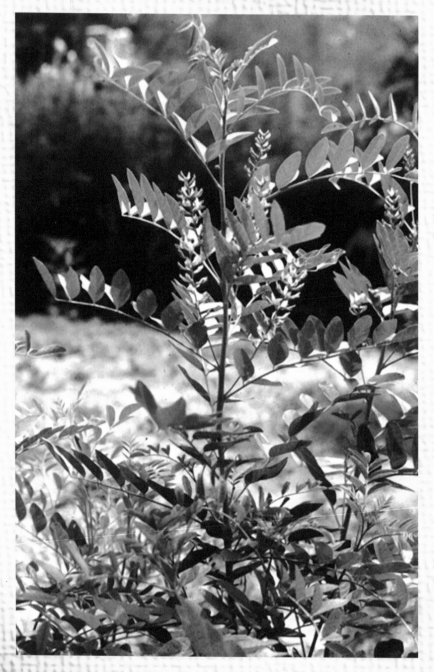

**Licorice**

ice creams and even beers where it also gives a darker color to the drink.

## PREPARATION AND DOSAGE

Decoction - although we can find Licorice pastilles at the pharmacy, you can make your own decoction of the herb which is very effective against cough and bronchitis. Put 30 grams of the dried root in two cups of water and boil it for about 10 minutes. You can drink 3 cups daily and it will soothe the throat and the pharynx.

Powder - powder is used against stomach or other peptic ulcers. Take a teaspoon three times daily.

Tincture - take 1-3 ml of Licorice tincture three times daily for colds and ulcers.

## SIDE EFFECTS

It is best to be avoided by people suffering from hypertension or kidney disease and also by pregnant women. In healthy people.

Licorice is considered to be a safe herb although large quantities of it may increase the blood pressure and cause palpitations or muscle weakness.

## HISTORY

We find Licorice in almost all ancient civilisations. The first report comes from Egypt during the 3rd century while at the same time Theophrastus mentions the remarkable properties of sweet Scythian root (Licorice) that relieved from dry cough and all pectoral diseases. The name Glycyrrhiza was actually given to the herb by Dioscourides, and is a compound of two words, "Glycys" which means sweet and "rhiza" which means root.

Licorice has also been used in Chinese medicine and is considered to be the second most widespread herb in China after Ginseng. In Europe the herb appears to be extensively cultivated during the Middle Ages in Germany and Spain.

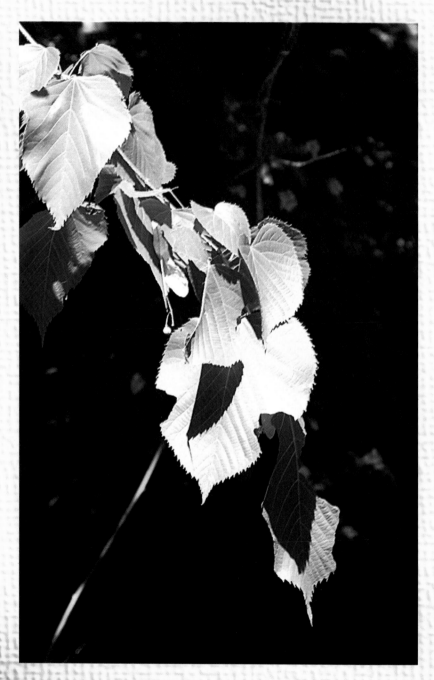

**Linden**

# Linden

*Nervine, astringent, anti-inflammatory,
emmenagogue, antispasmodic, diaphoretic*

**Scientific Name:** Tilia europea
of the Tiliaceae family.

**Parts Used:** leaves, flowers
and bark.

**USES**: Linden is used for the
treatment of:
- Headaches
- Migraine
- Rheumatism
- Arthritis
- Cystitis
- Constipation
- Indigestion
- Arteriosclerosis
- Hypertension

Linden is a relaxing herb suitable for problems of the nervous system. A decoction from the leaves of Linden will help people suffering from headaches and migraine. Its calming action and sedative effect can offer a lot of help to neurotic, hysteric and hypochondriac persons so it is widely recommended for everyday use to these people. Linden is a mild diuretic and as such it is very useful to people suffering from stones in the kidneys, cystitis and other problems of the urinary system. The bark of the tree is used for rheumatism, arthritis, dropsy, constipation, indigestion and even the blockage of the spleen or the liver. Its long-term use also protects from high blood pressure and the development of arteriosclerosis and sometimes it is used as treatment to people already suffering from the above diseases.

Linden is also used externally to reduce freckles and wrinkles of the face.

## PREPARATION AND DOSAGE

Decoction - boil 30 grams of Linden leaves or flowers or 4 teaspoons of the bark in a litre of water for two minutes and remove it from the fire. Leave it soak for another ten minutes and drain it. Drink 3 cups per day or use it externally on the face.

Infusion - soak 30 grams of leaves or two teaspoons of the bark in half a litre of water for five minutes. Drain it and drink 3 cups per day.

## HISTORY

The medicinal use of the leaves and flowers of Linden starts from the 18th century. Until then, herbalists limited their remedies only to the bark. However, there are some mentions of Linden in ancient times like the use of its leaves and the juice of the leaves as a poultice on snakebites, as Dioscourides suggests. Similarly, to emphasize its use against snakebites he says that snakes do not even dare to go near the Linden tree or its shadow. During the Second World War, when people were starving under the German occupation, people in France used to mix crashed dry leaves of Linden with Barley and Corn flour to produce what was known as "Green Flour" that was not really tasty but was nourishing and full of vitamins.

# Mallow
*Laxative, emollient, cleanser*

**Scientific Name:** Malva silvestris of the Malvaceae family.

**Parts Used:** leaves, flowers and root.

**USES**: Mallow is used for the treatment of:

- Bronchitis, cough, laryngitis
- Intestine problems
- Wounds and burns
- Ear infections

The root of Mallow is used internally to relieve from lung and throat pains while in large quantities it is used as an antioxidant, cleaning the organism from toxicities. Mallow is also used externally as a poultice or in salves for the cleaning of the skin and the fast healing of wounds and burns.

## OTHER USES

If we rub fresh leaves of Mallow on the area bitten by insects, it will relieve from the pain and prevent swelling.

## PREPARATION AND DOSAGE

Infusion - soak 20 Mallow flowers in a litre of water for about one hour and drink 3-4 cups daily.

Decoction - boil a handful of Mallow root in a litre of water for ten minutes and drink two cups daily. We can also use the leaves and the flowers instead of the root and if we want to use the decoction externally we have to double the quantity in the

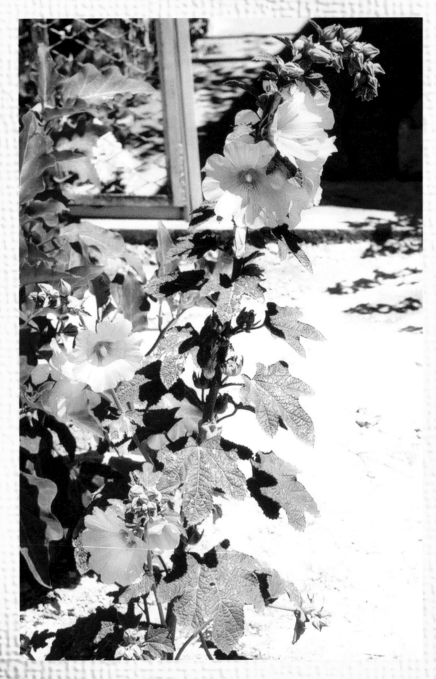

**Mallow** 166

same amount of water.

## HISTORY

There are scripts that prove that Mallow was known from 700 B.C. while for ancient Greeks it was a symbol of modesty and temperance. The students of the great Greek philosopher Pythagoras thought of it as a sacred plant because its flowers always turn towards the sun.

# Marjoram (Sweet)
*Tonic, emmenagogue, stomachic*

**Scientific Name:** Origanum marjorana of the Labiatae family.

**Parts Used:** leaves.

USES: Marjoram is used for the treatment of:
- Stomach gases and pains
- Headaches
- Insomnia
- Stress

Marjoram is used externally on bruises and wounds. Its volatile oil is used for soothing rheumatism pains while internally it is considered to be an excellent emmenagogue and a tonic in cases of weakness.

## OTHER USES

Marjoram is used as an aromatic in the kitchen and also used to aromatise closets and other spaces in the house.

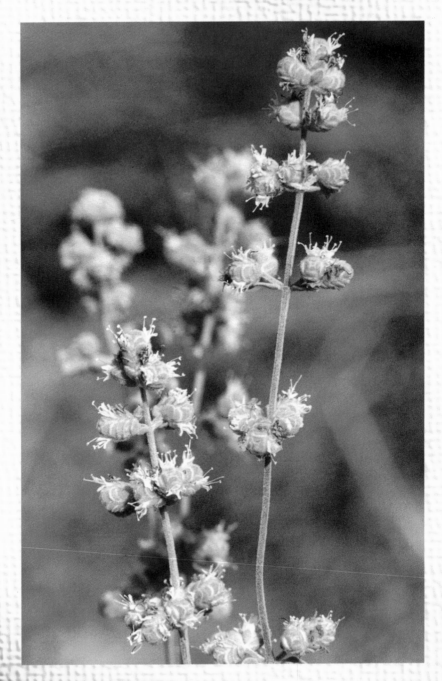

**Manjoram (sweet)** 168

## PREPARATION AND DOSAGE

Decoction - boil two teaspoons of Marjoram leaves in one cup of water for ten minutes and drink three cups daily.

Oil - use the oil externally or internally diluted in some water.

## HISTORY

Marjoram was well known in the old days and its origin is believed to be the Middle East. It was then exported to the Mediterranean countries and later on to the rest of the world. It was used by the Arabs and the Egyptians as a curative herb and according to Theophrastus its properties were also known to ancient Greeks. Singers used to drink its decoction - and they still do-in combination with some honey to keep their voice clear.

# Marshmallow

*For cough, inflammations and sores.*

**Scientific Name:** Althea officinallis of the Malvaceae family

**Parts Used:** Root and leaves.

**USES:** Marshmallow is used as a treatment for:

- Dry cough
- Bronchitis
- Laryngitis
- Inflammation of the pharynx and the intestines
- Gingivitis, inflammation of the gums
- Mouth sores

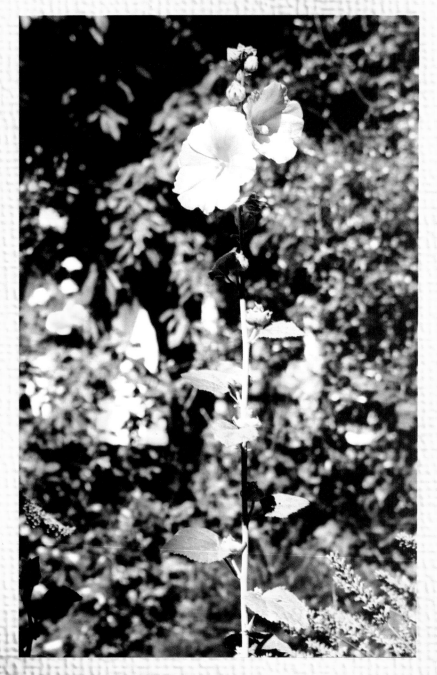

**Marshmallow** 170

Marshmallow is probably the best herb for diseases related to inflammations of the peptic system (especially the roots of it are very effective against mouth infections, sores, gingivitis, stomatitis) and infections of the peptic system (gastritis, colitis, intestine ulcers etc). The leaves of Marshmallow are very sedative to the irritated throat during winter cold and cures cough, pharyngitis and bronchitis. The tea of Marshmallow leaves is very good during a cold while the same tea is used as a diuretic and against gall bladder stones.

## PREPARATION AND DOSAGE

Tea for cough, bronchitis and inflammations - boil one teaspoon of dried leaves or flowers of Marshmallow in one cup of water for 1 to 2 minutes. Drain the leaves and flowers and cover the cup for ten minutes. It is not tasteful at all so it is better to sweeten it with some honey. You can drink it three times a day.

Cold Infusion - Put 2-4 grams of Marshmallow root in a cup of cold water and leave it to soak for one night. The infusion can be used for mouth diseases, gall bladder stones and as a diuretic.

## OTHER USES

The root of Marshmallow is used to add flavor to certain alcoholic drinks and syrups.

## HISTORY

Dioscourides refers to the therapeutic properties of Marshmallow against hug and intestine diseases and also mentions the use of its flowers in funerals. The Chinese used the roots of the herb for food and they still do while a lot of historians refer to Marshmallow at periods of famine and starvation.

# Milk Thistle

*Liver supporting, antioxidant, cholagogue, appetizer, tonic.*

**Scientific Name:** Silybum marianum of the Compositae family.

**Parts Used:** Leaves, flowers, stem, seeds.

**USES:** Milk Thistle is used for the treatment for:
- Liver diseases
- Gall bladder stones
- Psoriasis
- Spleen problems

Milk Thistle is considered to be protective to liver cells, protecting them from dangerous toxins and even regenerating injured cells. The leaves are often used for minor stomach problems like dyspepsia or bad appetite. The seeds are used to treat gallstones, spleen problems, jaundice and gallstone colic. It is also used as an antidote to mushroom poisoning.

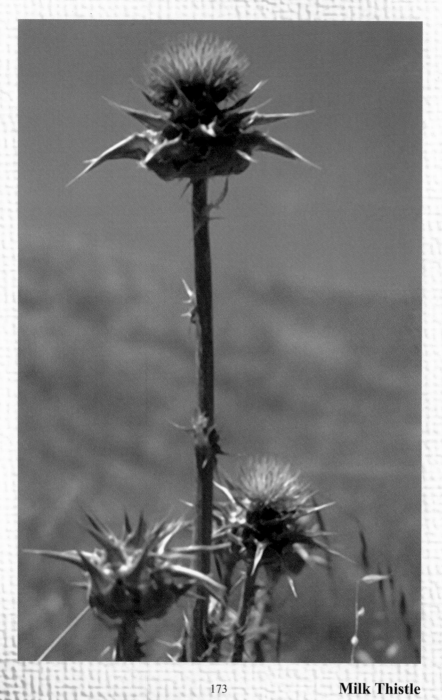

173 **Milk Thistle**

## PREPARATION AND DOSAGE

Decoction - boil 30 grams of Milk Thistle seeds in one litre of water and drink up to 3 cups per day. You can boil 50-100 grams of seeds in a litre of water if you need a stronger decoction.

Tea - put 30 grams of dried Milk Thistle in one litre of hot water. Leave it for ten minutes, drain it and drink one cup, three times a day.

Standardised silymarin - ask your pharmacist for a herbal extract of Milk Thistle standardized to 70%-80% of silymarin. Patients with liver anomalies should take about 400 mg of silymarin daily reduced to 200 mg daily in two months. Your doctor of course will provide all necessary instructions.

## OTHER USES

The dried leaves of Milk Thistle mixed with some water, are used to increase the milk flow to nursing mothers. People who suffer from hemorrhoids can sit for 15 minutes in a mixture of dried leaves and water.

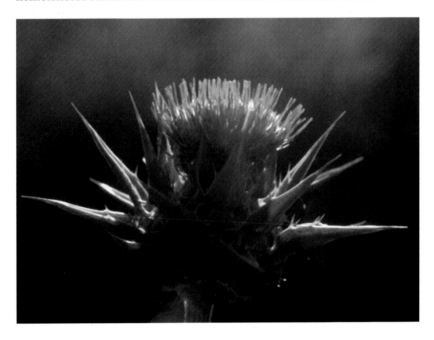

## SIDE EFFECTS

The dosage mentioned above should be strictly followed because too much Milk Thistle may cause vomiting. On the contrary, large quantities of Milk Thistle are often deliberately used to provoke vomiting to people that have been poisoned, to empty their stomach.

## HISTORY

Milk thistle was used - and it is still being used - as an antidote to Amanita phalloides (know as the death cap mushroom) which destroyes the liver cells and eventually causes death to the victim.

Dioscourides, the famous Greek botanologist mentions that the seed of Milk Thistle was given to people bitten by serpents and also to infants that have their sinews drawn together.

On the other hand, Pliny, the Roman naturalist that lived in the first century A.D. refers to Milk Thistle as an excellent remedy for the restoration of liver functions. Although a lot of centuries have passed from the days of Dioscourides and Pliny, the use of Milk Thistle has not changed much, even today.

# Mustard

*Digestive, laxative, rubefacient, stimulant, emetic*

**Scientific Name:** Sinapis alba of the Cruciferae family.

**Parts Used:** seeds and its fresh leaves.

USES: Mustard is used for the treatment of:
- Indigestion
- Chronic constipation
- Colds, bronchitis and influenza
- Headaches
- Bruises
- Muscular and skeletal pains

175

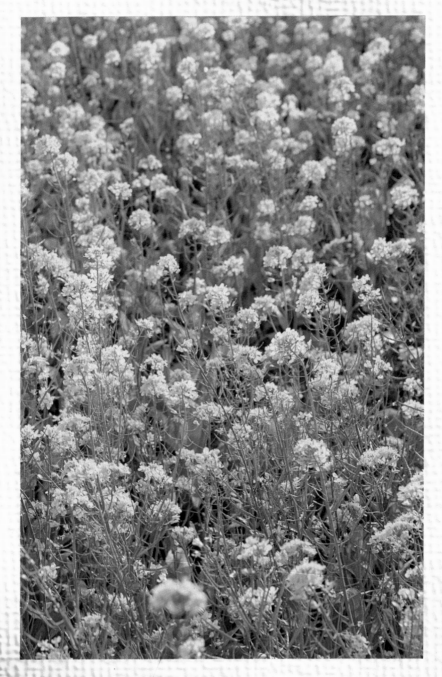

**Mustard** 176

There are three main species of Mustard: the white, the black and the wild. The white Mustard seeds have rubefacient properties and stimulate all the functions of the organism so their use gives a reviving feeling. The black Mustard has a pungent smell and is only used externally as a stimulant and emetic.

A decoction of the seeds of white Mustard is very effective for indigestion, chronic constipation and chronic bronchitis. Using it for gargles it relieves the sore throat.

The seeds of black Mustard are used always externally. Applying them at the area in pain as a poultice will promote blood circulation and relieve muscular and skeletal pains and of course rheumatism, neuralgias and pneumonia. It is also used on bruises.

For fevers, colds and flu, Mustard can be very helpful in tea form or in the bath.

**OTHER USES**

During the cold periods you can spray some Mustard powder in your socks. This will promote blood circulation and hyperemia providing warmth and energy. This is not recommended for an extensive use because it may increase the blood pressure.

Singers sometimes use a mixture of white Mustard powder in honey, early in the morning to keep there voice clear.

The boiled leaves and stem of Mustard are used in cases of flu.

## PREPARATION AND DOSAGE

Infusion - put one teaspoon of white Mustard powder into a cup of boiling water and leave it for five minutes. Drink three cups per day. Do not use more powder than the recommended quantity because it may cause intestine inflammations.

Poultice - crash some black Mustard seeds, add a few drops of water to form a thick paste. Place it in a piece of cloth and apply the poultice on the right area.

Bruises - mix some crashed black Mustard seeds with honey and apply the mixture on bruises to get rid of them and relieve you from pain.

Decoction - you can make a tea with white Mustard seeds boiling half a teaspoon in a cup of water for two minutes. Drink as much as three cups a day.

## SIDE EFFECTS

Do not consume undiluted Mustard seeds or powder because it is caustic and will cause severe intestine and stomach problems. Its essential oil is also very caustic and if used directly on the skin, undiluted, it will cause burns.

## HISTORY

Mustard has been cultivated in Europe since the Middle Ages and was used both for medicinal purposes as well as for preserving food because of its ability to induce  bacterial action. Today it is mostly known as a sauce but it is widely used in pharmacopoeia.

# Nettle
*Styptic, astringent, haemostatic, hair tonic,
anti-asthmatic, rubefacient, hypotensive*

**Scientific Name:** Urtica dioica
of the Urticaceae family.

**Parts Used:** the whole herb (its
stings are destroyed when the
herb is boiled or dried).

USES: Nettle is used for the
treatment of:
- Weakness
- Asthma
- Arthritis
- Hemorrhage
- Rheumatism
- Eczema
- Gall bladder stones
- Ague
- Cystitis
- Hemorrhoids
- Falling hair

Nettle has the property of diluting uric acid, a property that makes the herb useful in cystitis and gall bladder stones. In some cases of arthritis and rheumatism the Nettle has achieved remarkable results. It is hypotensive and this is why it is recommended to people that try to avoid salt since Nettle contains a variety of minerals and natural salts that do not harm the organism.

It is used both externally and internally for haemorrhages like nose bleeding and uterine bleeding (internal bleeding). Nettle has also been employed externally for the treatment of various kinds of eczema. For even better results on the treatment of eczema, Nettle can be combined with Figwort. The root combined with the herb helps in chronic rheumatism while the juice of the roots is employed to relieve from lung diseases like asthma and bronchitis. Young Nettles and Nettle juice are considered to be hair tonic and that they stimulate hair growth.

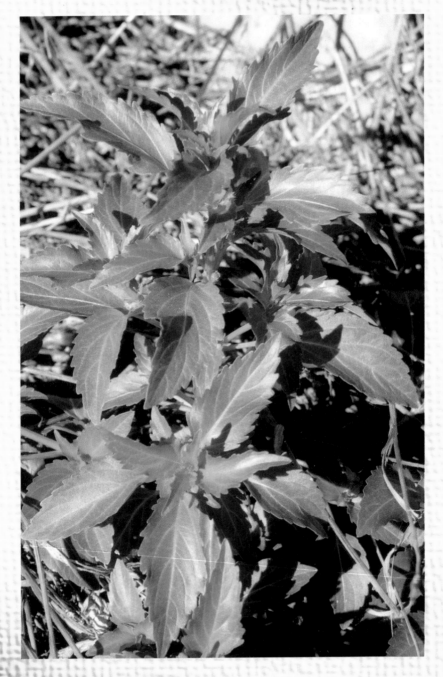

**Nettle** 180

## OTHER USES

Most animals except the donkeys will not eat fresh Nettle. If however, the Nettle is dried in the sun, its stings and the poison it contains are destroyed and it can be mixed with hey to feed cattle and sheep. It is a proven fact that cows fed with dried Nettle produce more milk. Similarly, if the Nettles is dried, finely chopped and used in poultry, a higher egg production is achieved with chickens. It is also used to fatten chicken and turkeys. Nettle is also used as a tonic to weak horses or as a digestive aid to horses suffering from peptic problems. It can be mixed with their food.

## PREPARATION AND DOSAGE

Infusion - soak 2-3 tablespoons of crashed leaves of the root in a cup of water for 10 minutes. Drink three cups per day.

Decoction - boil one handful of the herb or the root, or a combination of both in one litre of water for 3 minutes. Remove it from the fire and leave it to soak for another twenty minutes before draining it. Drink three cups daily. The same decoction can be used for gargles for mouth wounds and abscesses. For chronic rheumatism, boil one handful of the herb or the root in a litre of water for ten minutes and drink the whole decoction in 6 doses, in between the meals.

Syrup - mix the juice of the roots with honey or sugar until the mixture becomes smooth and homogenous. Take one tablespoon, three times daily to relieve asthma or bronchitis.

Hair tonic - gather a handful of young Nettle and simmer it in a litre of water for about two hours. Drain the Nettle and massage the scalp with the decoction every other night to induce falling hair and to revive the brightness and softness of the hair.

Powder - crash the roots and the aerial parts of the herb until they become fine powder and take 5-6 grams three times a day.

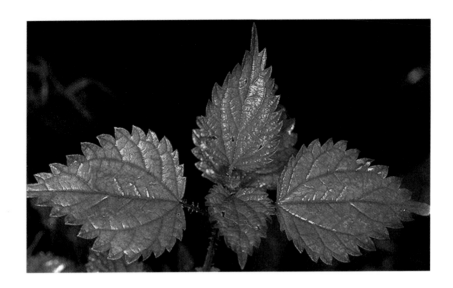

## SIDE EFFECTS

No side effects have been reported for using Nettle. Care should be taken however during gathering because of its stings. If you get stung by Nettle, just rub the area with Rosemary or Sage leaves and the itching will go away.

## HISTORY

Although not highly esteemed, the herb and some of its curative properties were known for thousands of years now, as these were mentioned by Pliny and Dioscourides. The Nettle was used as a medicine but it was also eaten when boiled and even used as a substitute for cotton in cloth making. The ancient Romans used the Nettle for the treatment of a lot of diseases and its use was eventually spread to all the countries under the Roman empire.

# Nutmeg

Antiseptic, stimulant, carminative, expectorant, digestive, aromatic

**Scientific Name:** Myristica fragrans of the Myristicaceae family.

**Parts Used:** seeds.

USES: Nutmeg is used for the treatment of:
- Indigestion
- Poor appetite
- Gallstones
- Bad breath
- Flatulence
- Nausea and vomiting
- Teeth neuralgia

In small quantities, Nutmeg is used internally for indigestion, flatulence, gallstones and the dilution of gallstones. It is used for the stimulation of the brain and the circulatory system and has been used for freshening the mouth and avoiding bad breath. Externally it is being used to relief from rheumatic pains and teeth neuralgias.

## OTHER USES

It is used in perfumes and cosmetics and is widely used as a spice in the kitchen.

## PREPARATION AND DOSAGE

Decoction - boil one teaspoon of Nutmeg powder in a cup of water for ten minutes, drain it and drink it. For external use we can

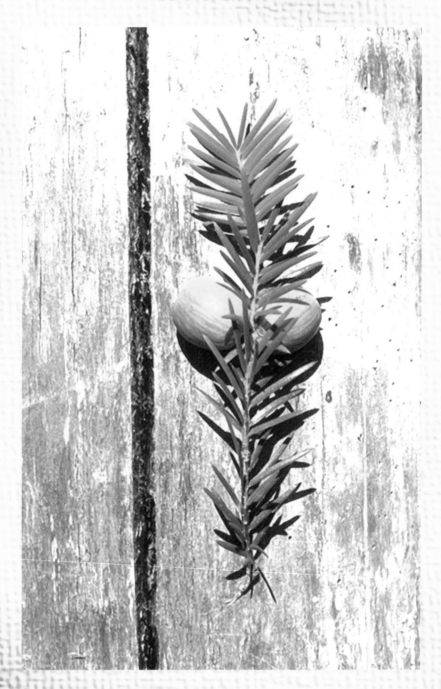

**Nutmeg** 184

use a stronger decoction or we can buy Nutmeg butter (salve) from the pharmacy.

## SIDE EFFECTS

Nutmeg has hallucinogenic properties which, as the name implies, may create hallucinations. In addition it may be the cause of stomach pains, double vision and delirium and in large quantities it will cause poisoning. Eating only two Nutmegs can be fatal. On the other hand, it should be avoided by pregnant women because one of its ingredients, Myristicin, provokes the onset of birth.

## HISTORY

Nutmeg is not growing in Europe and is actually a tropical evergreen tree native to Indonesia. From the Roman time, Nutmeg was used as a narcotic and later on as a spice. It is now being cultivated in a lot of tropical countries due to the big demand of both the spice and its volatile oil.

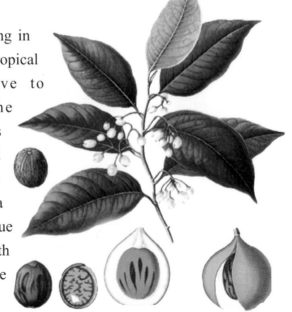

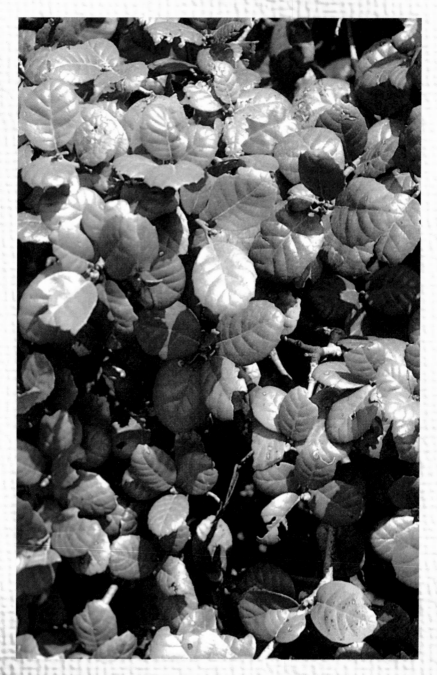

**Oak Tree**

# Oak Tree

*Antiseptic, astringent, anti-inflammatory*

**Scientific Name:** Quercus Orobus of the Compuliferac family.

**Parts Used:** The leaves, its bark and the fruit (acorns).

**USES:** Oak tree is used as a treatment for:

- Blood bleeding
- Hemorrhoids
- Tonsillitis
- Diarrhea
- Dysentery
- Cocitis
- Laryngitis
- Pharyngitis

### PREPARATION AND DOSAGE

Decoction - put one teaspoon of Oak tree bark in one cup of water. Warm through at a low temperature for 10 to 15 minutes and drink one cup three times daily. You can use the same decoction for external use on bleeding wounds or skin infections.

Tincture - Take 1-2 ml three times daily.

### HISTORY

Acorns were widely used in the past as food for the pigs but they were also eaten by people in rough times. In ancient Greece the Oak Tree was very sacred due to the fact that it was devoted to Zeus, the father of all Gods, and oak forests were strictly protected.

The Oak tree was also worshiped in ancient France.

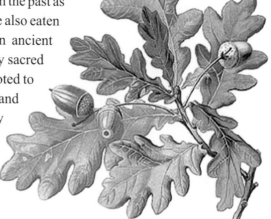

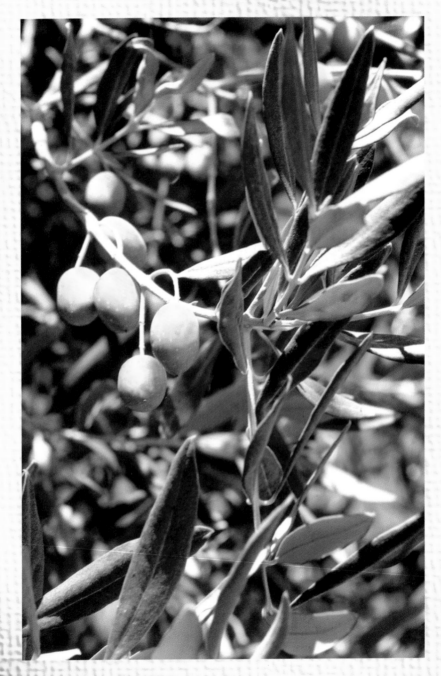

**Olive**

# Olive

*Astringent, antiseptic, laxative,*
*reduces cholesterol and triglycerides.*

**Scientific Name:** Olea europea of the Oleaceae family.

**Parts Used:** Leaves, bark and fruit.

**USES:** Olive or olive oil is used for the treatment of:
- Fever
- High blood pressure
- High Cholesterol levels
- Constipation
- Wounds and skin cracks

The decoction of the Olive leaves is a good antiseptic and is also used to reduce fever. A combination of the leaves with Lavender makes an effective sedative. Scientific studies have confirmed that virgin olive oil helps in reducing cholesterol and triglycerides levels in the blood. Externally, the olive oil is used to relieve from wound and scratches pain as well as insect bites. The decoction of the fresh bark of the tree reduces the blood pressure.

**OTHER USES**

As we all know, olive oil is extensively used in cooking and salads especially in the Mediterranean countries.

It is also used in soap production and as a hair tonic when combined with alcohol.

## PREPARATION AND DOSAGE

Oil - We can find plenty virgin olive oil in the market. For external use we just heat it slightly and use it always tepid.

Decoction - boil for 20-30 minutes 100 grams of olive leaves (or 50 grams of fresh bark) in a litre of water for ten minutes and then cover it until it cools down. For hypertension drink one cup of the cold decoction of the bark after each meal. For fever, drink 3-4 cups of the decoction daily. For high cholesterol or constipation swallow a tablespoon of virgin olive oil before each meal.

## HISTORY

The Olive tree held always a high position in the ancient world and still enjoys similar respect today. As we read in the Bible, Moses exempted from military services all men working in Olive cultivation. Olive oil is still considered sacred somehow and is used extensively in religious places all over the world to light lamps. The oil has through the ages become a symbol of kindness and purity and the leaves symbolise peace and happiness. During the ancient Olympics in Athens, the winners were crowned with a wreath of Olive branches.

# Onion

*Antiseptic, anticoagulant, anti-scorbutic, aphrodisiac*

**Scientific Name:** Allium cepa of the Liliaceae family.

**Parts Used:** bulb.

**USES:** Onion is used for the treatment of:
- Diabetes
- Staphylococcus
- Hypertension
- Rheumatism/arthritis
- Biological and mental exhaustion
- Prostate / impotency
- Infectional diseases

Onion has so many healing properties that they can only be described in a whole book but here we will cover only the most important ones. It's a strong appetizer and is used in cases of anorexia because it stimulates the digestion process (it must be avoided by people suffering from stomach diseases though). The fresh juice of onions is used by diabetics to reduce their blood's sugar level.

Anticoagulant - it reduces blood pressure, prevents thrombosis and in cases of anemia it provokes blood production.

Anti-rheumatic - raw onion is helpful to people suffering from rheumatism and arthritis.

Cleanser - it provokes perspiration, expelling toxins from the body, improves the digestive function of the intestines, cleans the intestines and expels undigested food.

Aphrodisiac - the reason for which it is considered to have aphrodisiac action is maybe due to the fact that it improves all the functions of the body.

Onion is used in homeopathy for the treatment of many diseases.

## OTHER USES

If your nails seem to break very easily, you can use onion juice on them that will make them stronger. Of course the smell is not so pleasant but you can

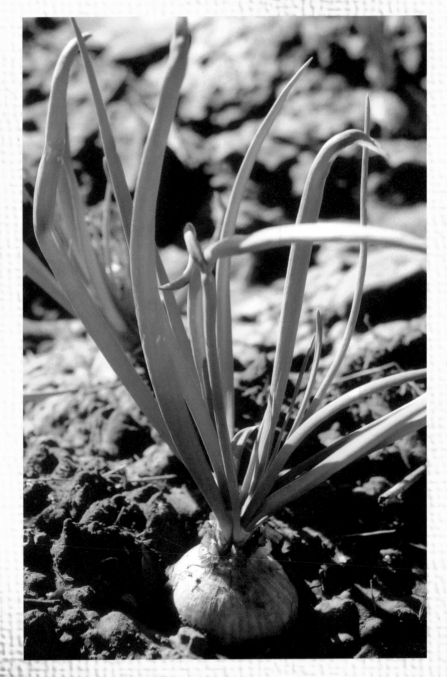

**Onion** 192

get rid of it by rubbing your hands with lemon and saltwater after using the onion. And similarly if we want a clean breath after eating onions, just chew some Peppermint or Parsley leaves.

Onion juice is also known as "invisible ink". If we write on paper using onion juice instead of ink, our writings can only be read near the fire or using the iron.

We admire magicians putting lighted candles and fire in their mouth. Before they do that they gargle with the decoction of dry Onions so that their mouth does not burn.

## PREPARATION AND DOSAGE

Infusion - Slice two big red Onions and place them in a litre of water. Leave them for one day and drink one cup, three times a day, for three or four days continuously.

Poultice - place raw Onion thickly sliced on the area you want to apply or use the thin membrane that separates the Onion leaves between them as a bandage.

Tincture - slice a raw Onion and leave it soaking into alcohol for one week. The alcohol must have the same weight as the Onion. We then filter the tincture and we take two teaspoons per day.

Foot bath - mince one big Onion and use it in one litre of water to put your feet in.

## SIDE EFFECTS

The only side effect you will have eating Onions or drinking its juice is the unpleasant smell, but of course there are ways to get rid of it as we have described above.

## HISTORY

Onions were definitely known in ancient China, Egypt and Greece. A lot of ancient writers mention the use of Onion as a medicine like Homer, Herodotus, Dioscourides, Theophrastus and Pliny. Its origin has never been concluded but it probably originated either from Persia or Afghanistan. Today Onion is used mostly as a spice or for food rather than as a medicine.

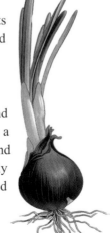

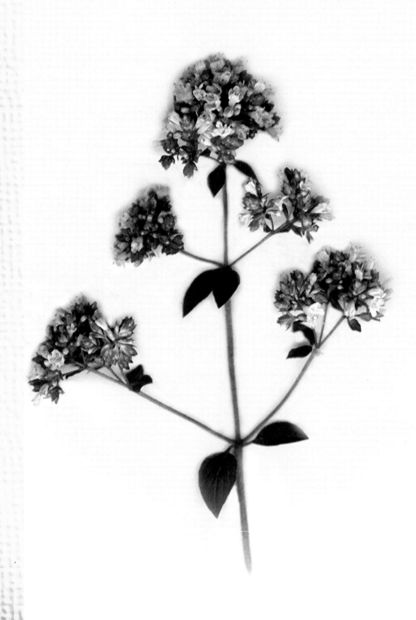

**Oregano** 194

# Oregano

*Tonic, stimulant, appetizer, astringent*

**Scientific Name:** Origanum vulgare of the Labiatae family.

**Parts Used:** flowering herb.

USES: Oregano is used for the treatment of:
- Stomach pains
- Diarrhea
- Intestinal problems
- Rheumatism
- Toothache

Oregano is valuable for many stomach problems and especially gastric weakness. Used internally, it will stop diarrhea, fight gases and flatulence. It is used for muscle pains, lung diseases and is especially helpful in chronic bronchitis. Its antiseptic properties make it useful in cases of tuberculosis of the lungs and asthma.

It is used as an astringent for intestine affections and pains in the stomach.

For women, it is considered to be emmenagogue in cases of menstrual period delays but it does not provoke abortion.

Used externally, it helps for wound healing and is used as an analgesic in muscle pains and arthritis.

## OTHER USES

Oregano has a calming and tonic effect when used in the bath.

It is widely used as a spice, especially on grilled

195

meat.

## PREPARATION AND DOSAGE

Decoction - boil one tablespoon of Oregano in a cup of water for 10 minutes. Drain it and drink three cups daily, one cup before each meal.

Infusion - soak one tablespoon of Oregano in a cup of hot water for 10-15 minutes.

Oil - use 3-4 drops of volatile oil of Oregano in a tablespoon of honey. Take it two to three times daily.

## HISTORY

Ancient Greeks knew of the medicinal action of Oregano for thousands of years and they used it internally (as a decoction) for poisoning, spasms and colic pains. Externally it was used to relieve from muscle pains and swellings. Oregano was - and still is in some places used by hunters on their hunting to keep it from smelling.

# Parsley

*Expectorant, carminative, emmenagogue, that has the property to reduce blood pressure.*

**Scientific Name:** Petroselinum crispum of the Umbelliferae family.

**Parts Used:** leaves, roots and seeds.

USES: Parsley is used for the treatment of:
- Kidney stones
- Hypertension
- Palpitations
- Menstrual pains
- Flatulence

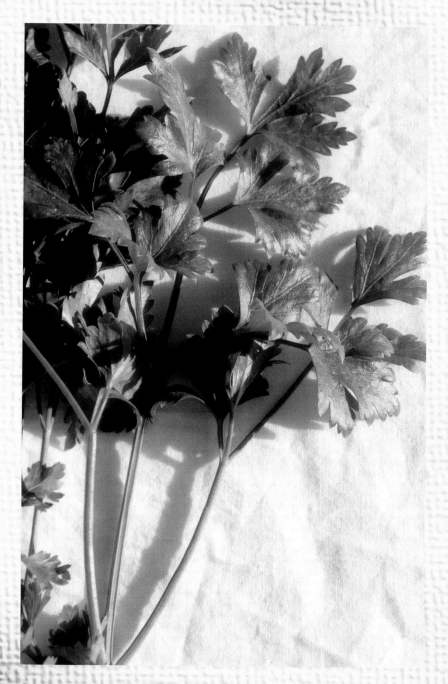

197 **Parsley**

Parsley has been used over the ages for many medicinal purposes but it has been highly esteemed for its diuretic properties and its curative action on the kidneys. A strong decoction of the root or the dry leaves of Parsley is excellent for treating gravel, kidney stones, congestion of the kidneys and jaundice. Parsley tea, prepared using dried leaves is very soothing in flatulence, colic pains and other stomach problems.

Parsley is also very helpful to women with troubled menstrual period. It is considered an effective emmenagogue and soothing for menstrual pains. Care should though be taken during pregnancy because it may cause an excessive stimulation of the womb that may even result to miscarriage.

An oil extracted from Parsley seeds, known as Apiol, is currently being used for all the problems mentioned above as well as for reducing high blood pressure and palpitations of the heart.

**OTHER USES**

Parsley is of course widely used in salads, soups and sauces. Another use of Parsley is drinking its decoction on a daily basis to provoke abortion.

**PREPARATION AND DOSAGE**

Decoction - There are a lot of ways to take Parsley, the easiest one being the tea which is prepared by boiling two teaspoons of dry Parsley leaves or finely cut fresh leaves in a cup of water for five minutes. Leave it to soak for 20-30 minutes and drink it. The roots of Parsley give a stronger decoction than the leaves. Boil 100 grams of Parsley roots in one litre of water and leave it to cool down. Drink two cups of it daily after each meal. It is good for digestion, diuretic and soothes the pains of the intestines and the stomach. We can get similar results if we use 20 grams of bruised seeds instead of 100 grams root. All the above decoctions are useful in kidney stones, hypertension, palpitations and menstrual pains.

## SIDE EFFECTS

Although Parsley is considered to be harmless, its use in large quantities either as a decoction or even in its fresh form may cause intestine bleeding, dizziness and slow heart beat. Its use is not recommended during pregnancy.

## HISTORY

A lot of historians and ancient physicians mention the curative properties of Parsley. In Greek mythology, Parsley was dedicated to Persephone while the ancient Greeks used to put Parsley in the graves of their dead to please the Charon. This tradition still goes on in some places, but this time Parsley is put in the graves to honor Saint Peter. Homer also mentions that Parsley was given as a tonic to the battle horses.

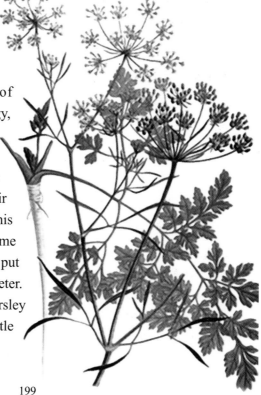

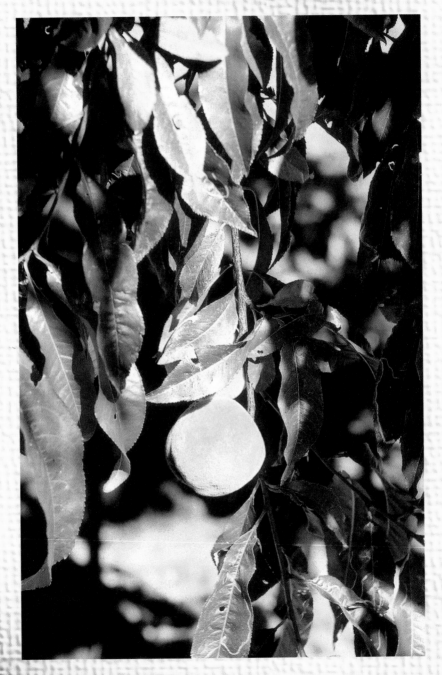

**Peach**                    200

# Peach

*Diuretic, sedative, expectorant, demulcent*

**Scientific Name:** Persica vulgaris of the Rosaceae family.

**Parts Used:** leaves, buds, flowers, kernels and bark.

**USES:** Peach is used for the treatment of:
- Stomach pains
- Arthritis
- Kidney diseases
- Burns, wounds and injuries
- Rheumatism
- Constipation

It is used internally for relieving from asthma, kidney problems and cystitis. It is a mild laxative for constipation. Its diuretic properties help people suffering from arthritis and kidney stones. It is also sedative and helps in insomnia. The leaves, the buds and the flowers are crashed and used as a poultice on burns, wounds and injuries. It stops bleeding and helps healing the wounds. The poultice is also used for colic, stomach pains and intestine problems. Compresses are used for itching and rheumatism.

## PREPARATION AND DOSAGE

Decoction - boil one or two teaspoons (depending on the age of the patient) of the leaves or the flowers of Peach in a cup of water for ten minutes and drink up to two cups daily. For cases of chronic bronchitis, boil 30 grams of the skin of peach in one litre of water and drink one tablespoon to one cup per day depending on the acuteness of bronchitis.

Syrup - mix the same quantity of Peach leaves, sugar and hot water until they become a smooth mixture. Let the leaves soak for two hours and drain the syrup. Use one teaspoon daily for children and one tablespoon daily for adults.

Peach juice - drink one glass of the juice in the morning with empty stomach.

Compress - boil half a handful of fresh or dried leaves for ten minutes and use this decoction on a cloth to make a compress.

## SIDE EFFECTS

Peach is a very good herb but we must take extra caution on the quantities we use because its flowers, leaves and especially the kernels contain small quantities of prussic acid that becomes poisonous at certain quantities.

## HISTORY

Although it may sound a bit strange, the Peach fruit was only lately used as food. In the past the Peach tree was cultivated, at least in Europe, for everything else than its tasteful fruit because it was considered suspicious. Although its scientific name Persica seems to be derived from the Greek "persica" meaning Persian, the tree's origin is not Persia (Iran) but China. Confucius mentions the use of Peach by the Chinese people.

# Peppermint
*Anti-inflammatory,*
*stomachic with sedative properties.*

**Scientific Name:** Mentha piperita of the Labiatae family.

**Parts Used:** Leaves and branches.

**USES:** Peppermint is used for the treatment of:
- Stomach pain
- Flatulence
- Intestine gas
- Cold / Flu
- Vomiting / Nausea
- Stress and overexcitement
- Menstrual Pain

Everyone knows of course that Peppermint tea is excellent for the cold and the flu. This herb has been used for centuries for stomach and intestine pain and disorders. It relieves from flatulence and promotes the production of digestive liquids in the stomach becoming very helpful in indigestion and colic pain. Its volatile oil acts as a moderate anaesthetic on the intestine walls making it very relieving in ulcers while at the same time it is used to fight nausea and vomiting, even to pregnant women or people that get dizzy when traveling.

## PREPARATION AND DOSAGE

Decoction - boil a teaspoon of Peppermint leaves in a cup of water for five minutes and drink it as often as you like.

Infusion - put 1-2 teaspoons of Peppermint

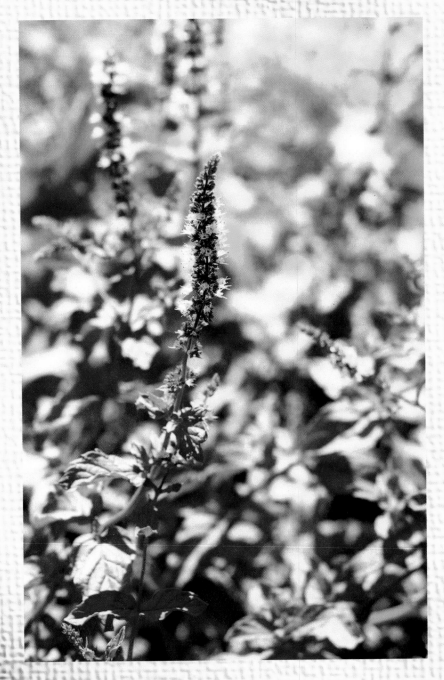

**Peppermint** 204

leaves in a cup of hot water. Cover if for 10-15 minutes and drink it.

Volatile oil - 1 to 3 drops in a cup of water

Tincture - 1 to 2 ml, three times daily.

## OTHER USES

Rats dislike Peppermint, a fact that can be very helpful when trying to catch rats in a house or keep them away. Use a rag soaked in peppermint oil.

# Pine

*Stimulant, tonic, diuretic*

**Scientific Name:** Pinus silvestris of the Pinaceae family.

**Parts Used:** the needle-like leaves and resin.

USES: Pine is used for the treatment of:
- Rheumatic affections
- Pneumonia
- Cough
- Depression
- Skin infections

Pine is used externally in salve form for rheumatism and in plaster form for bruises and sprains. Resin stimulates all glands and promotes all glandular action. Resin is used internally for acute bronchitis and pneumonia and disorders of the urinary system such as cystitis, gallstones and vaginal over secretion.

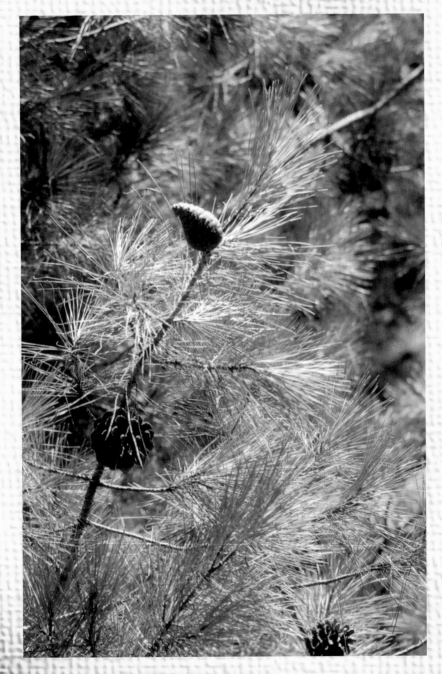

**Pine**

The decoction of the pine-nut is considered to be a fine tonic. The fresh yellowish buds are used in steamy water for inhalations in cases of bronchitis, cough and running nose. They are also used for colic pains and externally for various skin infections.

## OTHER USES

Resin is used in the veterinary practice as an antiseptic and diuretic. Resin is also employed in soap production and air fresheners.

## PREPARATION AND DOSAGE

Decoction - boil one handful of young, fresh leaves in a litre of water for 15 minutes. You can use this decoction externally in compresses or in the bath. For internal use, boil one pine-nut in half a litre of water for ten minutes and drain it. Add some honey to sweeten it and drink three cups daily.

Steam bath - boil for several hours some young, fresh leaves in a closed room (the bathroom may be of more convenience) and go in when the room gets steamy. For inhalations boil the fresh leaves with some yellowish young buds and pour the boiling water in the hot bath water. Get in the bath and inhale the steam.

## SIDE EFFECTS

People suffering from kidney diseases should not use Pine or resin.

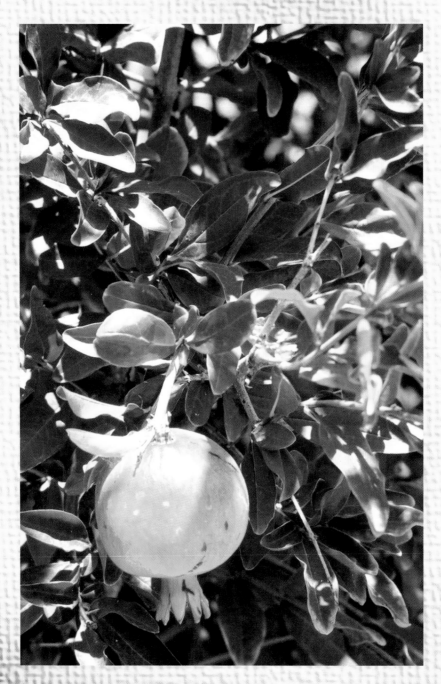

**Pomegranate** 208

# Pomegranate
*Astringent, sedative, aphrodisiac*

**Scientific Name:** Punica granatum of the Lythraceae family.

**Parts Used:** flowers, the skin of the fruit, fruits, bark and roots..

**USES**: Pomegranate is used for the treatment of:
- Stomach pains
- Diarrhea
- Dysentery
- Skin infections

The seeds of Pomegranate are analgesic, while the fruit itself was used in fevers and in cholera in the past. The skin of the fruit was used effectively in the past against intestine parasites like tapeworm. It is now being used in cases of diarrhea and dysentery and in India it is combined with opium for the same use. The decoction is used in cases of dysentery, the infusion is used as a gargle for sore throat and its powder is used for fever.

**PREPARATION AND DOSAGE**

Decoction - boil 30-50 grams of the fruit skin in one litre of water for 15 minutes. Drain it and drink three cups daily. If the skin of the fruit is dry, then soak it for 24 hours in water before you use it.

Tapeworm decoction - boil 60 grams of the skin of the fruit in one litre of water until half the quantity of the water is left. Before boiling the skin, soak it in the same water you will use later for 24 hours. This treatment must be combined with a strict diet and castor oil.

Poultice - boil some flowers or root in some water and apply them on the affected area of the skin.

Pomegranate is not recommended at any form to children under 5 years old, pregnant women and very nervous people. Big quantities may also cause vomiting.

### HISTORY

Pomegranate was considered to be the symbol of fertility. Even today, young girls hang the Pomegranate fruit on theirs necks in some places. Both Pliny and Dioscourides mention the curative properties of Pomegranate in their writings. As early as the first century B.C. Dioscourides recognized its property to fight parasites and specifically tapeworm.

# Poplar
*Fights fever and sore throat, tonic, diuretic*

**Scientific Name:** Populus nigra of the Salicaceae family.

**Parts Used:** bark, leaves and closed buds.

**USES:** Poplar is used for the treatment of:
- Fever
- Malfunction of the urinary system
- Stomach disorders
- Sore throat

The use of Poplar for medicinal purposes gives impressive results. The bark of the tree is recommended for high fevers and its diuretic properties make the herb useful for gonorrhoea and inflammations of the

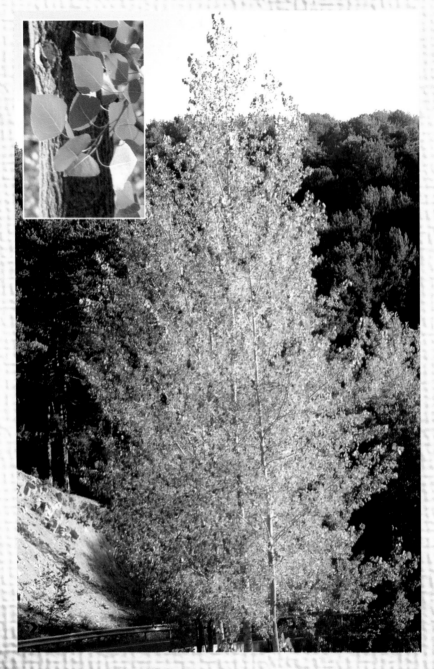

**Poplar**

urinary system. The decoction of its bark is used for the treatment of chronic diarrhoea and the decoctions of the young buds are excellent for rheumatism and arthritis. The decoction of the leaves helps in wound healing.

## PREPARATION AND DOSAGE

Infusion - place one teaspoon of Poplar buds in one cup of boiling water for 10 minutes. Drain it and drink three cups daily or even more until effect is achieved.

Decoction - boil two teaspoons of Poplar bark or three teaspoons of the leaves in a cup of water for 5 minutes and leave it to soak for ten minutes. Drink three times daily.

Tincture - 1 to 2 ml of the tincture, three times daily.

## HISTORY

In Greek mythology, Poplars were the sisters of Phaethon that were crying wildly, because of their brothers death. Zeus, not bearing to hear them cry, even though he killed their brother by lightning, transformed them into trees.

# Pumpkin

*Diuretic, laxative, wound healer, fights worms*

**Scientific Name:** Cucurbita maxima of the Cucurbitaceae family.

**Parts Used:** seeds, the flesh and the flowers.

**USES:** Pumpkin is used for the treatment of:
- Wounds and burns
- Skin rashes and cracks
- Nausea

Pumpkin is generally a balanced source of proteins, nourishing and energising. It is also a good source of iron, vitamin B and E, fibres and minerals. Pumpkin seeds are rich in Zinc, a mineral essential in wound healing which also helps in the treatment of enlarged prostate. They also contain many other useful minerals such as phosphorus, magnesium, copper, potasium, niacin, folic acid, pantothenic acid and others as well as unsaturated oils and antioxidants.

These nutritious seeds are also very good diuretics and expel parasites. They are used effectively to fight tapeworms and roundworms. A very important aspect of Pumpkin seeds is that they are completely harmless, they don't have any toxicity, therefore they can be safely given to everyone, even to small children.

Pumpkin oil and flesh will heal wounds and skin cracks.

The seeds but mostly the flesh of Pumpkin are used as a laxative and are considered to be very helpful in cases of constipation.

## PREPARATION AND DOSAGE

Poultice - grind several raw pumpkin seeds until they become pulp and use it as a poultice.

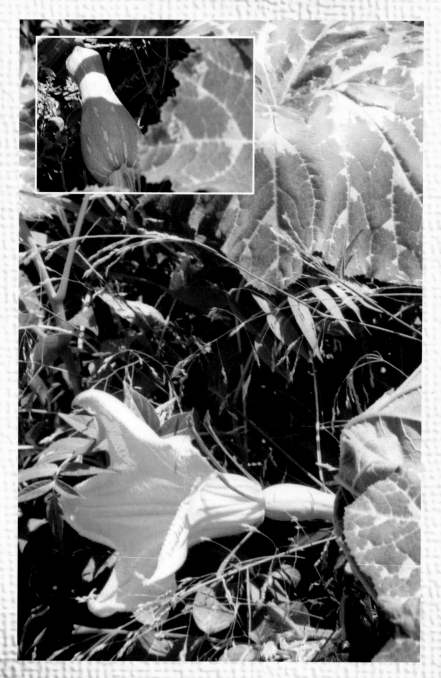

**Pumpkin**                    214

Laxative - boil 800 grams of pumpkin flesh with 200 grams of apples (sliced in small pieces) and 2-3 tablespoons of sugar in very little water. When they are heated into pulp, drain the water and give it to the person suffering from constipation to eat it. It may offer instant relief. (You can add a few drops of lemon just to improve its taste).

Parasites - peel 60-70 grams of Pumpkin seeds so that their shell is removed and put them in some hot water to get soft. Grind them slowly adding some drops of water while grinding until the mixture becomes a thick liquid, milky in color. Patients with parasites or even tapeworms should drink this mixture early in the morning, before breakfast.

*TIP* - You can store Pumpkin and its fresh seeds in a cool place away from insects but if you need to keep them for a long period you can use the fridge where you can store them for a long period without losing their properties.

## SIDE EFFECTS

Do not use Pumpkin flesh or seeds extensively because it may cause liver malfunction.

## HISTORY

Pumpkin was of great value to American Indians long before the Europeans arrived. The Indians were actually using Pumpkin both as medicine as well as for food and they were cultivating it extensively especially in Central America.

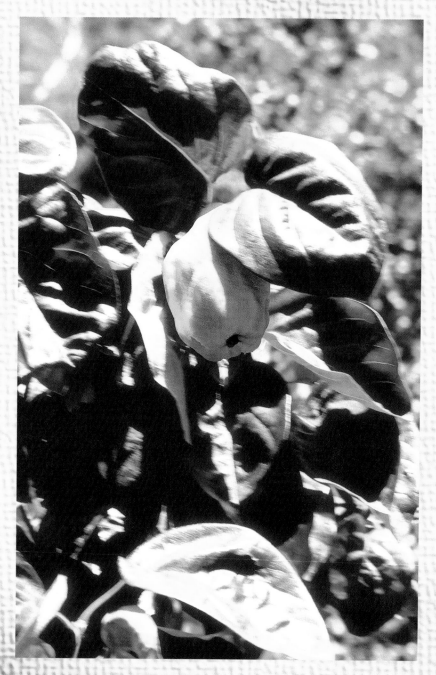

**Quince**

# Quince

*Expectorant, emollient, aphrodisiac*

**Scientific Name:** Cydonia vulgaris of the Rosaceae family.

**Parts Used:** fruits, leaves and seeds.

**USES:** Quince is used for the treatment of:
- Cough
- Sore throat
- Headache
- Insomnia
- Diarrhea, Dysentery, Vomiting
- Chilblain, skin cracks

It is used internally for diarrhea, dysentery and vomiting and as a decoction is recommended for cough, headaches and insomnia. As an infusion it is used in cases of constipation and intestine disorders.

It is also sedative in cases of nervous palpitations, insomnia and other problems of the nervous system. Quince has a lot of other medicinal uses such as for the soothing of sore throats, haemorrhoids (as a poultice) and even as an aphrodisiac for women.

## OTHER USES

Quince fruit is used for the production of wine, liqueurs, sweets and its essential oil.

## PREPARATION AND DOSAGE

Decoction - boil 25 grams of Quince seeds in one cup of water for ten minutes. Drink three cups daily for cough and headaches or one cup before going to bed for insomnia.

The same decoction can also be used for external use.

Infusion - soak 5 Quince leaves in 100 grams of distilled water. Use it for Chilblains, skin cracks and eye pain.

Poultice - boil a fruit until it gets soft and use it for hemorrhoids and headaches.

**SIDE EFFECTS**

The intake of Quince seeds is forbidden because they may cause vomiting.

**HISTORY**

The fruit of Quince was dedicated to Venus and it was a symbol of love and hapiness for ancient Greeks.

# Redclover

*Antispasmodic, emollient, tonic, expectorant, detergent*

**Scientific Name:** Trifolium pratense of the Papilionaceae family.

**Parts Used:** flowers and seeds.

USES: Clover is used for the treatment of:
- Anemia
- Bronchitis
- Cocitis
- Cancerous tumors
- Skin problems

Clover is one of the most effective treatments to a lot of skin problems in children. It can be safely used in cases of child eczema and has been combined with Nettle to treat other skin affections. It has been found very useful in cases of psoriasis, not only for children but also for adults. This property of red Clover is very significant due to the lack of any other effective treatment of chronic psoriasis using chemical medication.

Its antispasmodic and expectorant properties make it an excellent treatment for bronchitis, cough and especially whooping cough (cocitis). It is considered to be a blood purifier, that is why it is used in cases of anemia and some forms of cancer in combination with other herbs.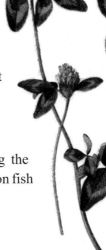

It is also used for anorexia and a fluid extract of red Clover is used as an analgesic.

## OTHER USES

A very tasty sauce can be prepared using the flowers of red Clover served as an appetiser or on fish and vegetable dishes.

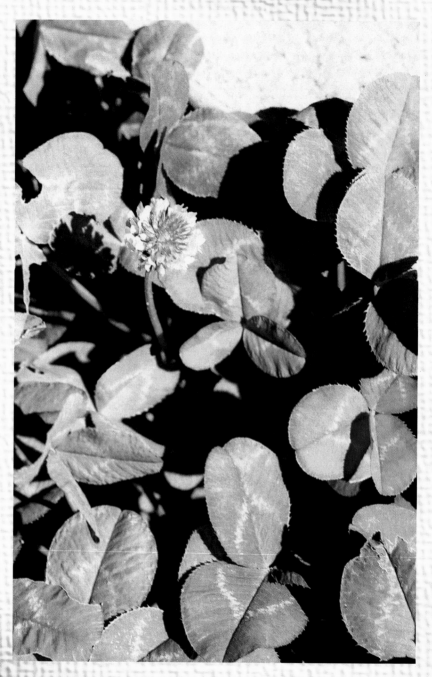

**Redclover**

## PREPARATION AND DOSAGE

Infusion - soak 2 teaspoons of dried Clover flowers in a cup of hot water for 15 minutes. Drain it and drink it three times daily.

Tincture - take 2-6 ml of the tincture, three times daily.

Decoction - boil two teaspoons of Clover flowers in a cup of water for ten minutes. Drain it and drink it three times daily or use it as a compress on cancerous growths, psoriasis and other skin problems.

# Rose

## *Tonic, astringent, diuretic*

**Scientific Name:** Rosa canina of the Rosaceae family.

**Parts Used:** rose petals.

**USES**: Rose is used for the treatment of:
- Headaches
- Dizziness
- Mouth abscesses
- Tonsillitis
- Mouth wounds

Rose is used internally mostly as an astringent for leucorrhoea, mouth abscesses, diarrhea and pulpy tonsillitis. It can also be used in gargle form to heal from mouth wounds and abscesses and the decoction of Rose petals has been used to soothe from headaches and dizziness. It is a very mild and pleasant herb and this is why it is recommended for children.

Externally, the decoction or the infusion of Rose petals is used to wash irritated eyes. Women suffering with menstrual pains may find Rose petals in their bath very relaxing.

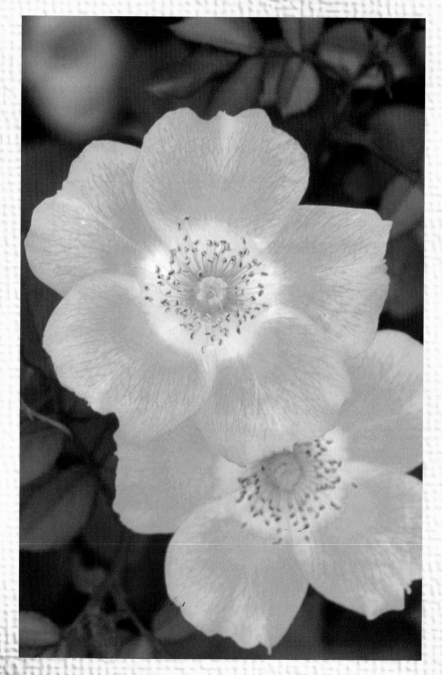

**Rose**

222

## PREPARATION AND DOSAGE

Infusion - soak one tablespoon of Rose petals in a cup of boiled water for ten minutes. Drain them and drink three cups daily, after each meal.

Syrup - soak one cup of Rose petals in half a litre of hot water for 24 hours (It is better if we keep it near a fire or at least at a warm place). Drain the petals and put the infusion on low fire, adding 300 grams of sugar. Stir it until it becomes a smooth syrup and remove it from the fire. Take 2-4 tablespoons daily.

Rose-honey - put five handfuls of dried Rose petals in a litre of hot water and leave them soak for 12 hours with the pot covered. Drain the petals and add 750 grams of honey while the infusion is warming on low fire. Keep stirring the mixture, removing the foam on top until it becomes a homogenous syrup.

Wash and gargles - soak 2 teaspoons of dried Rose petals in a cup of hot water for 10 minutes and then drain the petals. Use it for washing the irritated eyes or for gargles for mouth wounds and abscesses.

## HISTORY

There must be no place on earth where Rose has not been the symbol of love, gratitude, respect, etc. There is almost a story for it, any place you go. In ancient Greek mythology, the rose grows because of the nectar of the Gods that was accidentally dropped on earth by the small God Pothos (meaning lust) while he was dancing. For Christians it is a symbol of purity and as such is devoted to Mother Mary. For Islam, the Rose grew at the places where Mohamed's sweat fell on earth. There are hundreds of stories and myths that praise the beauty of Rose and describe it as a symbol of eternal love and devotion. The young wife of Toutanhamon, the ancient Egyptian Pharaoh that died in young age, wanted to show her love and devotion to her husband by placing a bouquet of Roses in his tomb. The Roses were found almost untouched by time, 30 centuries later.

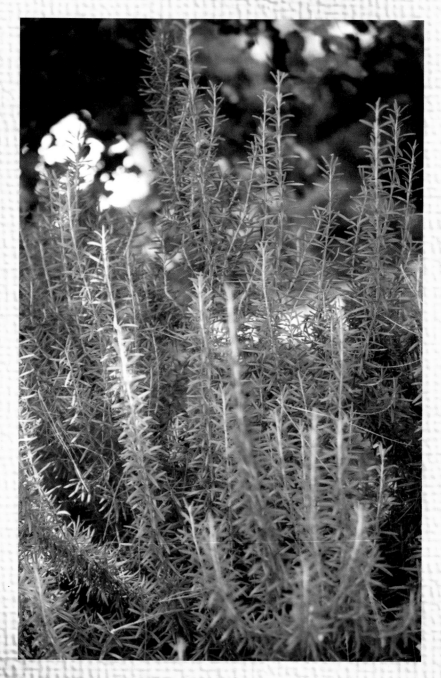

**Rosemary**

# Rosemary

*Tonic, antiseptic, antidepressant, sedative*

**Scientific Name:** Rosmarinus officicinalis of the Labiatae family.

**Parts Used:** leaves, roots and the flowering tops.

**USES:** Rosemary is used for the treatment of:

- Arthritis
- Diarrhea
- Depression
- Heart weakness
- Neuralgia headaches
- Dandruff
- Flatulence
- Falling hair
- Fatigue

It is used externally to relief from muscle pains, neuralgia, sciatica (pain in the hips) and bruises. It is used as a stimulant and promotes blood circulation to the head. It also stimulates the hair glands inhibiting falling hair. In some places it is the basic ingredient of remedies that fight baldness.

Even today, it is being used in some hospitals as an air cleanser and antiseptic. They burn Rosemary leaves in combination with cypress leaves to keep the air clean and fresh.

Internally, it is used to promote blood circulation, to strengthen the heart and stimulate the nerves. On the other hand it is used to fight stress and mild to moderate depression. It can also be very effective when used for indigestion, diarrhea and colitis.

It is used as a menstrual aid and in some places it is used to discontinue pregnancy.

## OTHER USES

Rosemary wine drunk in small quantities acts as a heart tonic and relieves accompanying dropsy since it stimulates the kidneys.

The volatile oil of Rosemary is used in fragrances, beverages, cosmetics and sweets.

## PREPARATION AND DOSAGE

Decoction - put a small branch of Rosemary in a cup of water and boil it for 5 minutes to be drunk before dinner. Diabetics can drink a stronger decoction (two small branches in a cup of water) early in the morning before breakfast. You can also bathe with the same decoction to get relieved from nervous headaches.

Infusion - put 1-2 teaspoons of dried Rosemary leaves in a cup of hot water and leave it covered for 10-15 minutes. It can be drunk up to two times daily as an anti-diabetic, antispasmodic, sedative and digestive.

Wine - place a branch of fresh Rosemary (preferably with flowers) in a bottle of white wine and leave it for about one week. It is a good tonic of the brain, the heart and nervous system and also used to relieve from headaches caused from bad blood circulation.

Volatile oil - use 3-4 drops of the oil in one tablespoon of honey, two to three times daily.

## SIDE EFFECTS

We should always avoid taking large quantities of Rosemary, especially of its volatile oil. Use only recommended dosage because it may cause vomiting, nausea, loss of concentration and in extreme cases even death.

## HISTORY

It is sometimes called the "sea dew" due to the fact that it grows near the sea. In the past, young brides used to decorate their head with a wreath of Rosemary since the plant was a symbol of marriage and love. On the other hand, in some places it was a symbol of death and this is why it is found in some ancient tombs.

It also had the reputation of being the "elixir of life" and during the Middle Ages it was supposed to fight away all evil spirits.

# Saffron

*Emmenagogue, anodyne, appetiser,*
*expectorant, rejuvenative*

**Scientific Name:** Crocus sativus of the iridaceae family.

**Parts Used:** dried stigmas on the flowers and the roots.

**USES:** Saffron is used for the treatment of:

- Indigestion
- Asthma
- Anemia
- Depression
- Diarrhea
- Dysentery
- Menopause
- Menstrual disorders

It is used internally, always in small quantities only, for colds, flatulence and insomnia. Its decoction is useful in cases of respiratory diseases and in extreme cases of sudden changes of mood and depression. Saffron is sometimes used to soothe eye pain and menstrual disorders with dark and thick blood.

It is added to liqueurs where it acts as an appetiser and eases digestion. The salve produced from Saffron is used for the treatment of gout. Its sedative properties are employed against stomach and muscle spasms and ticks.

## OTHER USES

Saffron is used in perfumes and dyes.

## PREPARATION AND DOSAGE

Decoction - boil 10 grams of Saffron stigmas in one litre of water

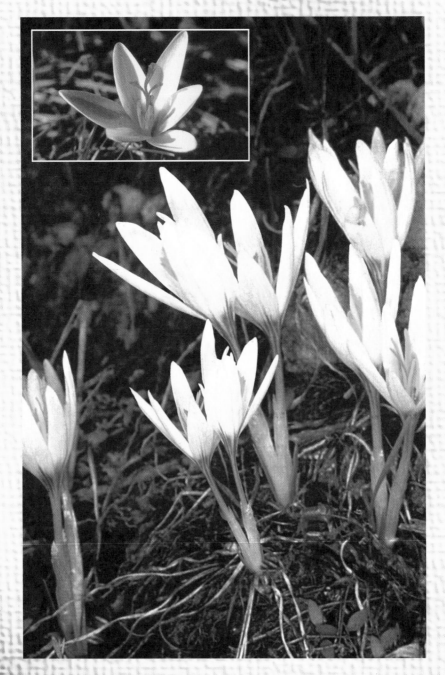

**Saffron**

228

until half of the original quantity remains. Drain it, add a little sugar and boil it again for 15 minutes. This will give us a syrup from which we can drink 2-3 teaspoons per day.

Infusion - soak 6-10 stigmas in half a litre of water for ten minutes and drink it for dysentery or diarrhea. Take half to one cup daily, a mouthful at a time.

Tincture - 5 to 15 drops daily.

## SIDE EFFECTS

Large doses of Saffron can have severe effects due to the fact that it contains poison that acts on the central nervous system and damages the kidneys. If the dose is high enough it can be narcotic and it can even be fatal in quantities exceeding 10 grams.

It is not recommended to pregnants.

## HISTORY

Saffron's name is derived from its yellow, coloring ingredient and comes from the Arabic word "za'faran" which means yellow. One gram of that ingredient can add color to 100 litres of water. It is non-fading and has been used extensively in icon painting. It was introduced to Europe by the Arabs and was known to the ancient Greeks and Romans. The price of Saffron is extremely high due to the fact that the valuable stigmas on the flower contain limited quantities of the active ingredient. More than 120,000 of flowers are needed to produce one Kilogram of Saffron.

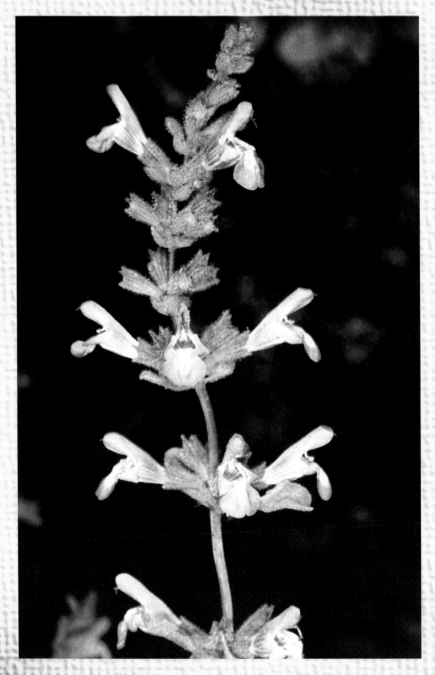

Sage

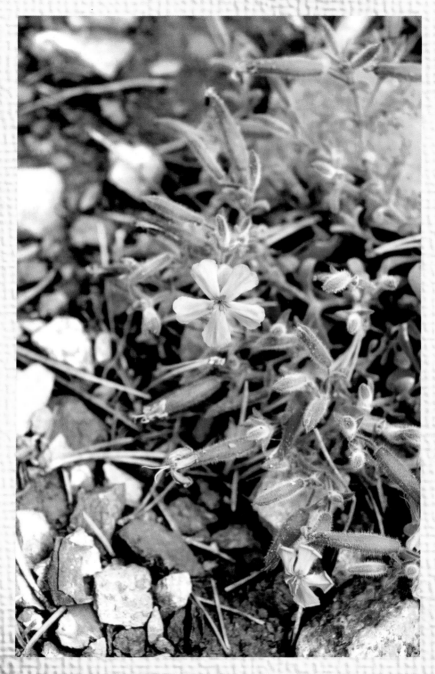

235                                    **Soapwort**

been proven useful for jaundice, indigestion and other intestinal disorders. As a tonic it is used to boost the kidney function and helps people with rheumatism and arthritis. The roots of Soapwort are used externally on a lot of skin affections including eczema, acme, skin cracks. It has a curative action on skin disorders caused by any form of syphilis.

## OTHER USES

Soapwort contains Saponin, a substance that is extracted to manufacture special soaps used for washing silk and wool clothes.

## PREPARATION AND DOSAGE

Decoction - boil 15 grams of Soapwort root in a litre of water for only two minutes and drain it instantly.

Infusion - put two tablespoons of finely cut root or 3-4 tablespoons of the leaves in a litre of hot water and leave it until it cools down and drain it.

Both the decoction and the infusion can be used internally and externally. A good remedy for external use is 70 grams of the herb's flowering tops in a litre of hot water until it cools down. It can be used for skin disorders as well as for falling hair.

## SIDE EFFECTS

Soapwort contains Saponin so care should be taken with its use.

# St John's Wort

*Antidepressant, tranquilizer, anti-inflammatory,*
*astringent, helps wound and burns healing,*
*fights anxiety and stress.*

**Scientific Name:** Hypericum perforatum of the Hypericaceae family.

**Parts Used:** Flowers and its tops.

**USED:** St John's Wort is used for the treatment of:
- Depression
- Skin inflammation
- Wounds and burns healing
- Anxiety
- Injuries
- Skin infections

Clinical trials have determined that St John's Wort can be as effective as the chemical antidepressants (like Prozac) in cases of mild to moderate depression. Compared though with chemical antidepressants, the side effects of St John's Wort are much less and more tolerable. The herb is also used internally for the treatment of bronchitis, asthma, spasmodic cough and collic pain.

Diuretic - it helps with problems of the cyst and anomalies of the urinary system in general.

Antiseptic - used for the treatment of insect bites, wounds and dysenteria.

Astringent - it helps wound and burn healing, and accelerates the elimination of leucorrhoea spots and skin tumors.


**PREPARATION AND DOSAGE**

Decoction - Put one teaspoon of finely cut flowers or leaves of the herb in a cup of hot water and leave it for about ten minutes. Drink 2-3

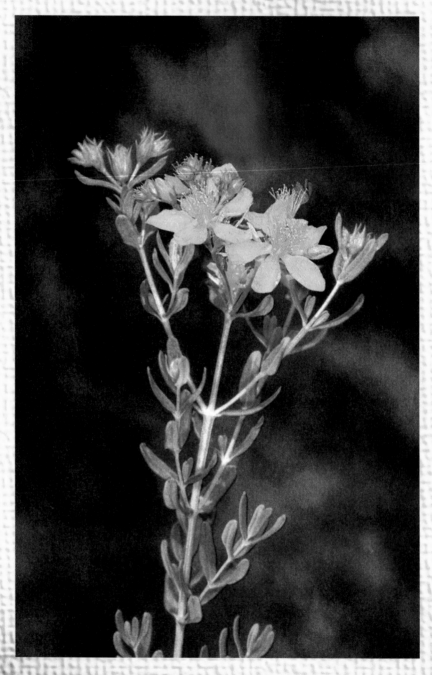

**St John's Wort**                    238

cups daily.

Extract - Put two teaspoons of the flowers of the herb in one cup of cold water.

Oil - mix some flowering tops with the herb's branches (10:1 ratio) in a litre of virgin olive oil. Close the bottle and leave it for 2-3 weeks, until the oil becomes red brownish in color. 5-10 drops of this oil in half a glass of distilled water relieves stomach aches, sourness and ulcers. Externally, this oil can be applied to wounds, burns, bruises and skin tumors.

Another use is filling your pillow with some leaves of the herb. Due to their calming fragrance, this will help people troubled with insomnia sleep better.

## SIDE EFFECTS

If the herb or any preparations of it are used very often it may cause vomiting or diarrhea.

## HISTORY

People in ancient Greece believed that the strong fragrance of St John's Wort had the power to cause the evil spirits to fly away. It is from this superstition that it derived its scientific name Hypericum, a Greek word meaning "above the spirits". At the same time, the ancient Greeks used to use it to fight depression and anxiety and externally for the healing of wounds, burns and even snake bites, uses that were also familiar all over Europe a few centuries ago.

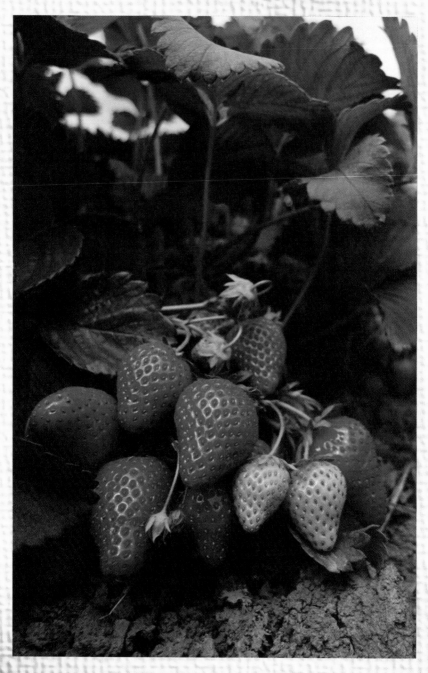

**Strawberry** 240

# Strawberry
*Laxative, diuretic, astringent, dentifrice*

**Scientific Name:** Fragaria vesca of the Rosaceae family.

**Parts Used:** leaves, root and fruit.

**USES**: Strawberry is used for the treatment of:
- Blood purification
- Constipation
- Fever
- Dysentery
- Diarrhea

Both the leaves and fruits of Strawberry are used in pharmacopoeia although the leaves are used more often. The fruits are easily digested and do not provoke acetous fermentation in the stomach. They contain malic and citric acids and are rich in vitamins useful for exhaustion. The roots of the plant have astringent properties and are used for diarrhea. The leaves possess similar properties and are used for diarrhea as well as for dysentery in tea form. The juice of the fruit has dentifrice properties and when the fruit is rubbed on the teeth it removes discoloration.

### PREPARATION AND DOSAGE

Decoction - boil one handful of Strawberry leaves or roots in a litre of water for twenty minutes. Drain it and drink it three times daily.

Skin cleanser - cut some fresh Strawberries in halves and rub them on the face right after you have washed it with hot water. This will open the skin pores and clean the face from dead cells and will also relieve from mild sunburn. In cases of heavy sunburns use the same technique as above but leave the Strawberry juice on the skin for half an hour before you remove it with hot water in which we have already added a few drops of Rosemary volatile oil.

## SIDE EFFECTS

Strawberry is considered very safe but allergic people should avoid Strawberry if they develop itches or skin rashes.

# Sunflower
*Expectorant, reduces cholesterol
and fights arteriosclerosis*

**Scientific Name:** Helianthus annuss of the Compositae family.

**Parts Used:** seeds

**USES:** Sunflower is used for the treatment of:
- Cholesterol
- Cough
- Areteriosclerosis
- Flu and cold
- Diabetes

Sunflower has expectorant properties which means that it is very helpful for diseases of the throat, the larynx, common colds and cough. The oil that is produced from the seeds is used as a preventive for arteriosclerosis and has also been found to reduce cholesterol. It also prevents the formation of kidney and gall stones and helps in the proper function of the reproductive system. Medical trials have also shown that Sunflower is sedative to the nervous system, it improves sight and reduces the pains from arthritis.

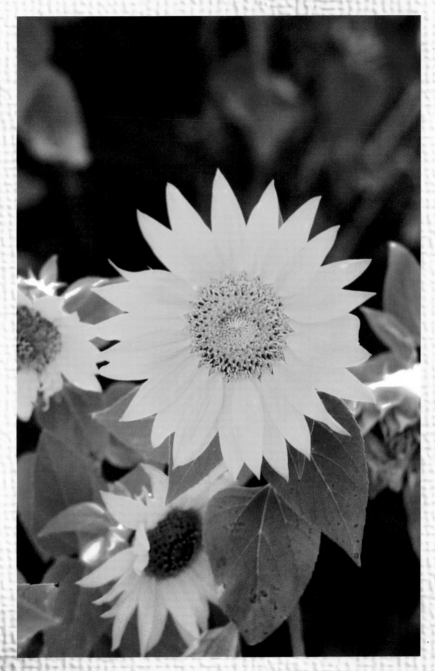

243 **Sunflower**

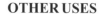

**OTHER USES**

Sunflower seeds can be used in certain appetisers, salads, bread and soups.

Raw Sunflower seeds are good for people on diet. Half a cup of raw seeds produce 280 calories.

**PREPARATION AND DOSAGE**

Infusion - put the Sunflower seeds in the oven until they become light brownish and then put two teaspoons in one cup of hot water for about ten minutes. Drink 3 cups daily to soothe whooping cough.

Oil - 10 to 15 drops of oil, two or three times daily.

# Thyme

*Antibacterial, carminative, diuretic, anti-spasmodic, sedative, stimulant, antiseptic, tonic, perspiratory*

**Scientific Name:** Thymus vulgaris of the Labiatae family.

**Parts Used:** leaves and flowering tops.

**USES:** Thyme is used for the treatment of:
- Anemia
- Digestion of fats
- Fatigue
- Blood circulation
- Menstrual pains
- Skin infections

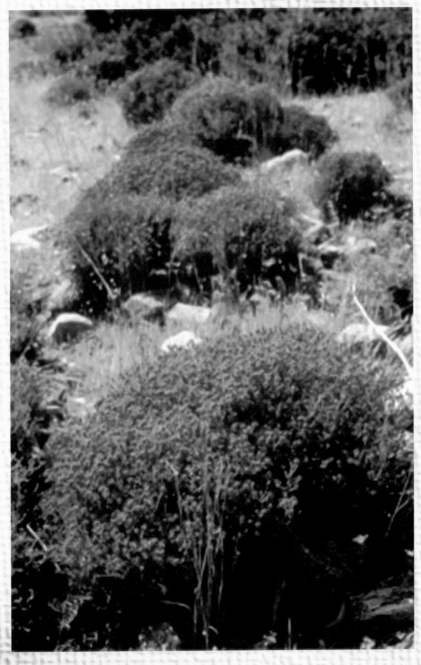

245

**Thyme**

Thymol contained in wild Thyme is extensively used for indigestion, especially for the sluggish digestion of fatty food. It is used as a tonic and stimulant, properties that make it an excellent remedy for stress, migraines, depression and other problems of the nervous system. It boosts the nerves and it is often used to people with low blood pressure as well as anaemic children. It is widely known as an antiseptic and is used both externally to prevent wound infections and internally to fight intestine infections, leucorrhoea, bronchitis and lung infections. It has also been used as a preventive antibiotic in flu epidemics and as a sleeping aid.

## OTHER USES

Thyme can also be used in the bath. Heat 500 grams of Thyme in 4 litres of water and mix it with the bath water. It is very good for people suffering from rheumatism, arthritis and even for common colds.

Thyme has the reputation that it may force an alcoholic person quit drinking making him disgust any alcohol. The remedy is quite simple: put a handful of Thyme in three cups of water. Leave it to soak for half an hour it and give to the alcoholic person, one tablespoon every 15 minutes.

Thyme is of course used in cooking, especially in fish dishes.

## PREPARATION AND DOSAGE

Decoction - heat a small branch in one cup of water. As soon as the water starts boiling, remove it and leave it to soak for 10 minutes. Drain it and drink one cup after each meal. It is very good in digestion but also effective in headaches, fatigue and other nervous infections. It can be combined with Rosemary.

Infusion - put two teaspoons of Thyme a one cup of hot water for ten minutes. Drink of this infusion three times daily.

External Use - cut the leaves in small pieces and warm them in very little water. Put it in a small piece of cloth and press on the infected wound with it.

Tincture - take 2-4 ml, three times daily.

## SIDE EFFECTS

Intake of large quantities of Thyme may result to thyroid over-function and even poisoning. Less serious symptoms of overdose are vomiting, diarrhea and dizziness.

## HISTORY

Theophrastus and Dioscourides mention the sedative and carminative properties of Thyme. Roman soldiers used to bathe in Thyme water to regain their strength, while, during the Middle Ages, women used to prepare Thyme arrangements for their soldiers to give them strength. Later on, Thyme was proved to be antibacterial against the anthrax bacillus and the bacteria of tuberculosis. Its antiseptic power is quite extraordinary, since the volatile oil of Thyme is 25 times stronger than Phenol.

# Valeriana
*Sedative, fights insomnia and stress.*

**Scientific Name:** Valeriana officinalis of the Valerianaceae family.

**Parts Used:** The whole plant but mainly the root.

USES: Valeriana is used as a treatment for:
- Insomnia
- Stress
- Epilepsy
- Hypertension
- Palpitations
- Nervousness

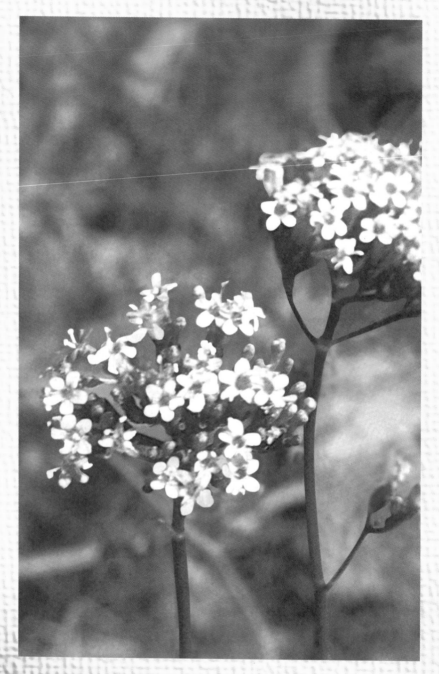

**Valeriana**

248

Valeriana has the incredible ability to reduce the stress and calm the nerves. Clinical studies have shown that people with insomnia problems had impressive results using Valeriana without having the side effects that sleeping pills usually have. Some researchers compare Valeriana favorably with Benzodiapezines like the widely known Valium. The big difference is that Valeriana is a "lighter" and safer sedative. Contrary to Valium and most other sedatives, Valeriana is not addictive and does not cause any dependence. In addition, its sedative properties do not change when combined with alcohol or other substances as benzodiazepines does.

Other clinical trials and animal experiments have shown that Valeriana can reduce blood pressure of hypertensive people. Valeriana has also shown that it may fight tumors and a lot of researchers believe that the herb or some of its ingredients may play an important role in curing cancer.

Another property of Valeriana is the positive effect it has on patients suffering from epilepsy. The herb is known to be antispasmodic and it reduces the heart pulse in cases of heart pulpitations. This is why Valeriana is so relaxing, relieving the organism from stress, anxiety and even neuralgia.

## PREPARATION & DOSAGE

Decoction - Put one teaspoon of Valeriana roots in a cup of water and leave it for 2-3 hours after you heat it for 10 minutes. You can drink a cup just before you go to bed.

Capsules - Take 300-500 mg of Valeriana root one hour before you go to bed to fight insomnia.

Children - Valeriana can be given to children too, but use half the above dosage.

Stress - 50 to 100 mg three times daily can relieve from mild stress.

Bigger dosage (300-500 mg, three times daily) can even replace chemical tranquilizers such as benzodiazepines (Valium etc).

## HISTORY

Dioscourides mentions Valeriana extensively in his books on herbs and recommends it for a number of problems like nausia, peptic deseases, liver problems and even anomalies of the urinary system. The calming and relaxing effect of the herb was known to people a lot of centuries ago. Valeriana was considered the most widely used treatment for neurological, even psychological problems until the 18th century.

The most widely known tranquilizer for many years now in Europe where someone will find more than 100 different preparations of Valeriana in pharmacies.

The herb is also found in Ayurveda where it is being used as a treatment of insomnia and for relaxation. For thousands of years Valeriana is also treated with the same significance in traditional Chinese medicine while in the USA it was widely used as a sleeping aid until the invention of the chemical sleeping pils, just before the 2nd World War. During the last decade there is a significant turn from chemical medicines to natural products.

# Vine
*Tonic, astringent, antiseptic, diuretic, cleanser*

**Scientific Name:** Vitis vinifera of the Viticeae family.

**Parts Used:** fruit and its juice, leaves.

USES: Vine is used for the treatment of:
- Gallstones
- Weakness
- Skin infections
- Hemorrhoids
- Diarrhea

Eating Grapes produces a lot of heat burning excess fat at the same time. Therefore, it is recommended to people who want to lose weight. Due to their diuretic property, they are also recommended to patients suffering from gallstones (gall bladder stones).

Astringent - the leaves of the Vine are used for diarrhea and hemorrhoids. They also regulate blood circulation, that is why they are used for the treatment of phlebitis, varicose veins, circulatory system disorders, menstrual period pains and menopause disorders. They are also used against hemorrhage when applied on wounds.

Red wine has a tonic effect while white wine is diuretic.

## OTHER USES

Grapes are used for weight loss. They work better if they are eaten in the morning with empty stomach. The recipe is quite simple: eat two Kilograms of grapes daily for the first time. If we eat the whole grape, including the pits, we might avoid diarrhea. The recipe should be avoided by old

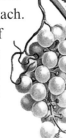

251

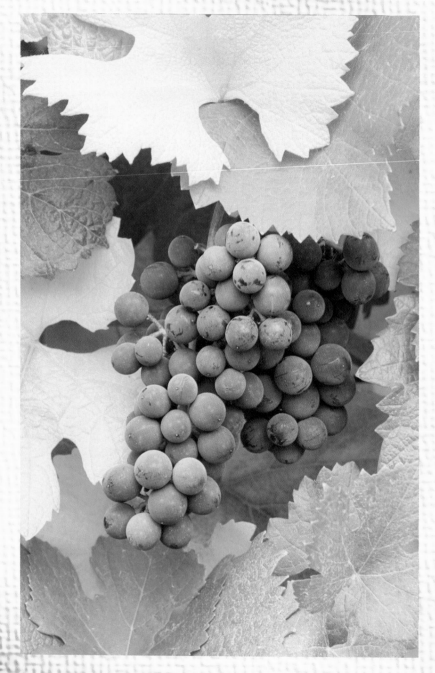

**Vine**

people that suffer from respiratory problems.

The seeds and the leaves are used in dry powdered form to treat dysentery in cattle.

## PREPARATION AND DOSAGE

Decoction - boil two tablespoons of finely cut Vine leaves in three cups of water for ten minutes. Drink one cup after every meal.

For external use, boil two handfuls of leaves for 15 minutes in a litre of water and use it in the bath.

Grapes - in cases of anaemia and exhaustion the restorative power of Grapes is striking. They are also useful in small-pox.

Raisins - raisins are dried grapes and are sold in the market. They are demulcent, nutritive and slightly laxative.

## SIDE EFFECTS

People suffering from diabetes or colitis should not eat Grapes especially the ripe ones. The same applies to Grape juice.

Excitable, full-blooded and dyspeptic people should avoid large quantities of ripe grapes because they influence the kidneys producing a free flow of urine and may cause palpitations.

## HISTORY

Vine was definitely used from ancient times both as fruit and for the production of wine. It is mentioned in the Old Testament that the patriarchs used to eat a lot of Grapes, and this might be the reason for their life longevity. Ancient Greeks dedicated the Vine to God Dionysus who taught them how to produce wine from it. Today, there are more than 3.000 types of vine cultivated all over the world.

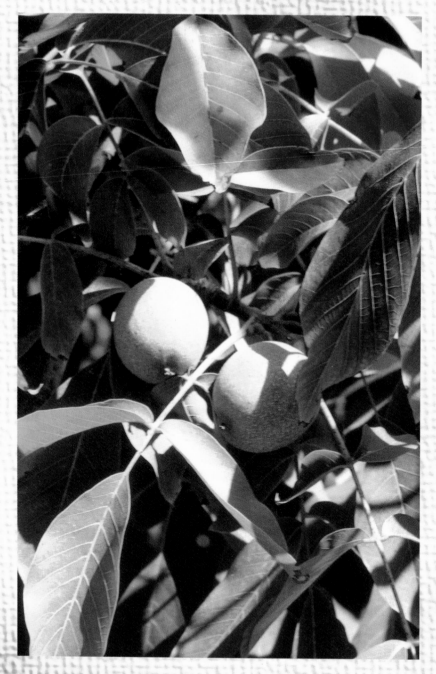

**Walnut**

254

# Walnut
## *Laxative, astringent, detergent*

**Scientific Name:** Juglans vegia of the Juglandaceae family.

**Parts Used:** leaves, flowers, fruit and bark.

**USES:** Walnut is used for the treatment of:
- Wounds and bleeding
- Diarrhea
- Leucorrhoea
- Colic
- Skin diseases

The leaves and the bark of the Walnut have detergent and astringent properties and are used to treat various skin diseases. The flowers can help people suffering from diseases of the glandular system, herpes, eczema and mild ulcers. Its juice is a blood purifier and small sprigs are used against falling hair and dandruff. The leaves and the flesh of the fruits are very astringent and contract the blood vessels making them useful for hemorrhoids, unusual bleeding during menstrual period, diarrhea and dysentery. The fresh leaves can be used in tea form to reduce the sugar levels of the blood and also against eye infections, abscesses and mouth sores. Finally, the unripe fruit has the ability to fight worms.

## OTHER USES
The Walnut oil, produced from the flesh of the fruit - the eatable part- is used in some places as an alternate to olive oil or butter and is said to have similar nutritional properties. The fresh walnuts (just before they become hard) are used to make an excellent sweet. The external peel of the nuts and its root are used for the production of cloth and leather paints. The leaves are insect repellants.

## PREPARATION AND DOSAGE

Decoction - Boil two handfuls of dry or fresh bark in one litre of water for 10 minutes and drink daily two cups of it. Alternatively, we can use 8-10 Walnut leaves in the same quantity of water.

Infusion - put 30 grams of dry bark or leaves in half a litre of hot water and leave them to soak for 6 hours before draining. Drink three cups daily. For a lighter infusion, put two teaspoons of dried Walnut leaves in a cup of hot water and drain it after 10 minutes. Drink 2-3 cups daily.

Compresses - put about 15 leaves in one litre of water and soak the cloth which you will use for compresses in it.

Bath/massages - two handfuls of fresh leaves or green bark in two litres of water. Use the water in your bath or for massaging on infected area.

## SIDE EFFECTS

No side effects are known for Walnut except that during gathering fresh nuts will leave a yellow greenish stain on your fingers which will eventually go away after several days.

## HISTORY

The Walnut tree is relatively new in Europe, and it is believed that it has been imported as late as the 16th century. Before that, it was only found in Greece and Near Eastern countries although its cultivation has now been expanded to many places around the world. It is believed that the most ancient recipe was found by Caius Pompeius when he discovered the treasury of Mithridates, the king of Pontus. A scroll of the latter's handwriting was found that was actually a recipe against any poison: take two dry walnuts, as many fresh figs as you can eat and twenty leaves of rue, bruised and beaten together with twenty juniper berries and some salt. Take it early in the morning to protect yourself from any poison or infection during the day.

# Watermelon
*Antioxidant, diuretic, antipyretic*

**Scientific Name:** Citrullus vulgaris of the Cucurbitaceae family.

**Parts Used:** fruit, seeds and the rind.

**USES:** Watermelon is used for the treatment of:
- Diseases of the urinary system
- Fever
- Difficulties in urination

The seeds of Watermelon have excellent diuretic properties and are also used for infections of the urinary system such as gravel, kidney stones, arthritis and rheumatism. The fruit is useful in cases of prostate and difficulties in urination, while in combination with its rind it is used for fevers. Still, its use must be limited and it must be consumed slowly in very warm climates especially by people living in colder climates.

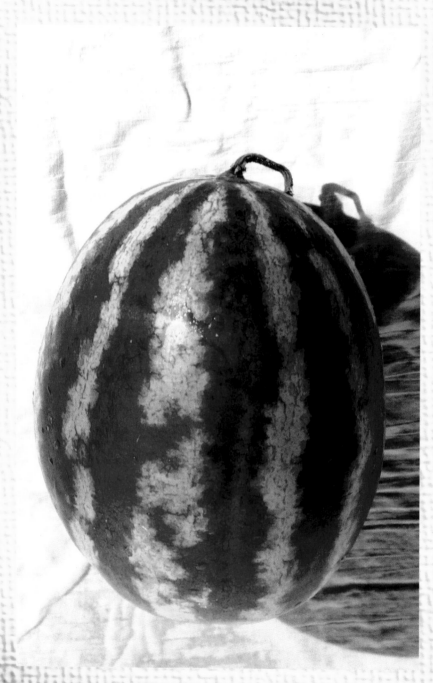

**Watermelon**

# Watermelon
*Antioxidant, diuretic, antipyretic*

**USES:** Watermelon is used for the treatment of:
- Diseases of the urinary system
- Fever
- Difficulties in urination

The seeds of Watermelon have excellent diuretic properties and are also used for infections of the urinary system such as gravel, kidney stones, arthritis and rheumatism. The fruit is useful in cases of prostate and difficulties in urination, while in combination with its rind it is used for fevers. Still, its use must be limited and it must be consumed slowly in very warm climates especially by people living in colder climates.

Watermelon has some of the properties of Pumpkin too. In some places it is being used to get rid of the intestine parasites, especially in small children.

## OTHER USES

Watermelon is of course one of the most refreshing fruits and it is being used as such. In some places its rind is being used for the production of a delicious and refreshing sweet.

The rind is also used in sunburns and relieves from eye inflammation.

## PREPARATION AND DOSAGE

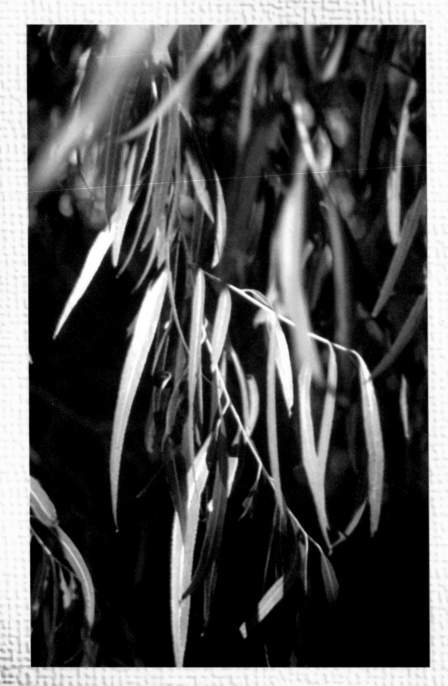

**Willow**

# Willow

*Antipyretic, tonic, analgesic, astringent, antispasmodic, anti-rheumatic, anti-inflammatory*

**Scientific Name:** Salix alba of the Salicaceae family.

**Parts Used:** leaves and bark.

**USES:** Willow is used for the treatment of:
- Inflammations
- Fever
- Headaches
- Arthritis
- Rheumatism

The antipyretic properties of Willow make it useful for colds and flu. It has similar to aspirin analgesic properties, although it is not as strong but still has longer effect. The bark of Willow is rich in Tannin and this is why it is recommended in cases of gastroenteritis.

## PREPARATION AND DOSAGE

Decoction - boil 50 grams of the leaves of Willow in one litre of water or a teaspoon of the finely cut bark in one cup of water. Boil it for one minute and leave it to soak for another 15 minutes before draining it. You can drink a cup of the decoction, three times daily.

## SIDE EFFECTS

Continuous intake of Willow is not recommended because it may cause the same side effects as aspirin. Nevertheless, Willow decoction is considered to be safer than aspirin.

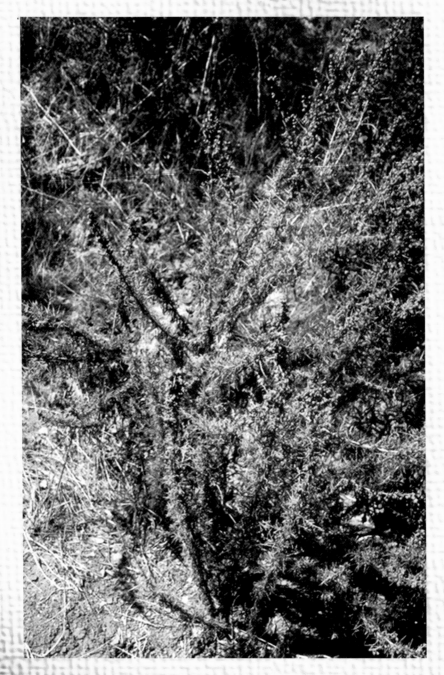

**Wormwood** 262

# Wormwood

*Digestive, Antipyretic, Spasmolytic.*

**Scientific Name:** Artemisia absinthium of the Compositae family.

**Parts Used:** the flowering tops, its leaves and roots.

**USES:** Wormwood is used as a treatment for:

- Anorexia
- Epilepsy
- Dizziness and fainting
- Diarrhea
- Liver insufficiencies
- Weight loss

It is used internally for digestion and intestine worms. It increases bile production and eases the digestion of fatty and oily food, that is why it is considered to fight indigestion and even helps people that want to lose weight. It fights epilepsy, especially some epileptic symptoms that occur to young teenage girls.

Wormwood is spasmolytic    stops spasms    especially to small children, in cases of dizziness and fainting. It is also used to strengthen the liver and to fight insomnia.

## PREPARATION AND DOSAGE

Decoction - Put 10 grams of the flowers in one litre of water and leave them for 15 minutes. Drain the flowers and drink it. The water may be warm or even cold and you can drink this or the tea of Wormwood for 3-4 days. It is advised to add some honey because the tea is quite bitter.

Another way to use Wormwood is by putting 25 grams of the leaves in one litre of white wine or beer and leave them in a closed bottle for two weeks.

## OTHER USES

Wormwood can be used as poultice to accelerate the flow of blood during difficult menstrual period. Put the poultices at the abdomen and combine this with a cup of Wormwood tea or decoction.

## SIDE EFFECTS

Wormwood is definitely a very good herb but it is advised not to drink it for a lot of days continuously because it may cause dizziness and headache. Pregnant and nursing women should not use Wormwood and the same applies for irritable people and people with stomach or intestine problems.

## HISTORY

Wormwood is mentioned in the Bible and its juice is described as bitter and thick and symbolises the difficulties of life. Its concentrated juice is in fact a very strong poison.

In very small quantities it may be served as an appetiser like ouzo. In big quantities it becomes a strong narcotic and is so addictive that you cannot quit it easily. The herb was known to the Egyptians, the Greeks and the Romans. It derived its official name from the ancient Greeks that devoted the plant to the Goddess Artemis, the Goddess of forests and hunting, and it was used by virgins to help their menstruation.

According to Avikenna, the Arab philosopher that lived during the 11th century, it was used as a good appetisers while three centuries later, medical students at the medical school of Salerno were treating a lot of deseases with Wormwood including nausea, cholera, jaundice, rheumatism and many others.

# Yarrow
*Appetizer, fights fatigue, antispasmodic, diuretic, antipyretic.*

**Scientific Name:** Achillea millefolium of the Compositae family.
**Parts Used:** All parts that grow above the ground especially its flowering tops and its leaves.

**USES:** Yarrow is used as a treatment for:
- Common cold / sore throat
- Thrombosis due to hypertension
- Eczema
- Hemorrhoids
- Indigestion
- Stomach irritations
- Small wounds
- Fever

Yarrow is one of the best perspiratives and is a widely recognised herb. The decoction of Yarrow helps the body to fight against fever. It lowers the blood pressure, helps digestion and strengthens the blood vessels. As an antiseptic it is given to people that suffer from infections of the uric system like cystitis. It is used as an astringent when used externally on wounds and is also used against hemorrhoids, breast nipple cracks, eczema, lichens, herpes and other skin problems. It is considered to be very effective to blood glotting due to high blood pressure. Experiments on animals have indicated that the specific herb can reduce muscle spasms.

It is also considered to be a blood purifier, this is why it is used to fight acme and herpes.

In women, it is used to soothe a lot of gynecological complications (dysminorrhia, aminorrhia, menopause anomalies, womb or uterus spasms). It also adjusts menstrual period.

## PREPARATION & DOSAGE
Boil one teaspoon in a cup of water or 25-30 grams in a litre of water for 10 minutes. Use it to wash the infected skin or wounds or to make compresses. We can also use the same decoction to stop falling hair.

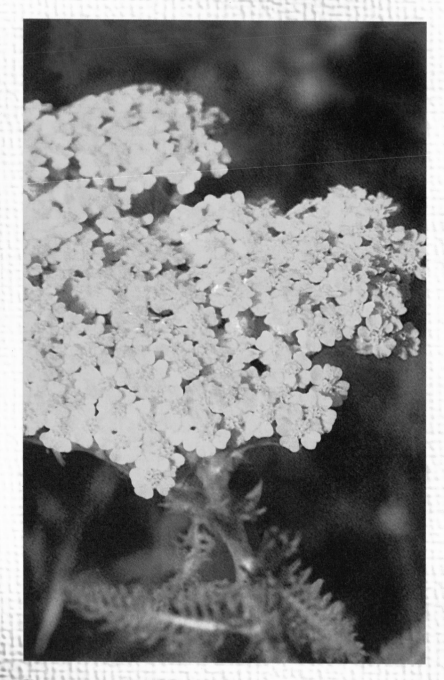

**Yarrow**

For common cold, we can inhale the steam produced when we boil 25-30 grams of Yarrow in two litres of water.

For hemorrhoids or for cleaning of an external skin wound boil 25-30 grams of Yarrow in one litre of water and use it (not very often because it may cause skin irritations).

We can drink the tea of Yarrow three times a day, except in fever situations when we can have it every hour until the fever drops. We can also use a Yarrow lotion externally, 2-4 grams three times a day.

## OTHER USES

The seeds of Yarrow are used as wine preservatives for wine stored in wooden barrels. It often replaces the hop used in beer manufacturing. It can also be used for body massage using a lotion of 10 grams of Yarrow essential oil, 20 grams of camphor lotion and 25 grams of lanolin.

## SIDE EFFECTS

Skin rashes or other allergic reactions have been reported in some cases so stop using Yarrow if you observe such reactions. The frequent use of the herb can also increase sensitivity to light. Be careful not to use it in deep or infected wounds. The use of Yarrow is not recommended during pregnancy and nursing.

## HISTORY

Yarrow millefolium got its name from Achilleas the Greek mythological hero - who after being wounded by Paris's poisoned arrow during the Trojan War, the Goddess of love, Aphrodite, revealed the herb to him and advised him to wrap it around his wound to heal it. Even today, Yarrow is considered to be very effective to wounds created by iron or steel objects. Dioscourides was also using the herb as haemostatic (to stop the blood bleeding) a treatment that was used even during the First World War by soldiers.

267

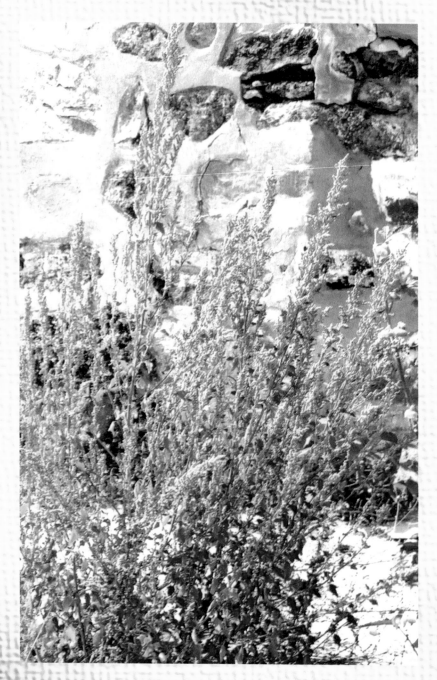

**Yellow dock**

# Yellow dock
*Tonic, cleanser, diuretic*

**Scientific Name:** Rumex crispus of the Polygonaceae family.

**Parts Used:** the whole herb.

**USES:** Yellow Dock is used for the treatment of:
- Skin infections
- Indigestion
- Anaemia
- Diarrhea
- Dysentery

Yellow Dock is extensively used for the treatment of chronic skin infections like psoriasis, herpes, eczema and scab. The roots are used as a tonic and have the property of increasing the appetite and fight anaemia by purifying the blood. The use of the whole herb has been employed to fight diarrhea, dysentery, diabetes, jaundice, hepatitis and hemorrhoids.

## PREPARATION AND DOSAGE

Decoction - boil 30 grams of finely cut roots or two handfuls of flowers in one litre of water for ten minutes. Drink 2-3 times daily, one cup at a time. We can use the same decoction externally.

Poultice - crash the fresh leaves or the root of Yellow Dock and use them directly on the skin.

## HISTORY

Yellow Dock was one of the most highly esteemed plants in the old times. It was also used in cooking and physicians of the 16th century considered the herb magical for infections, fevers and even poisoning.

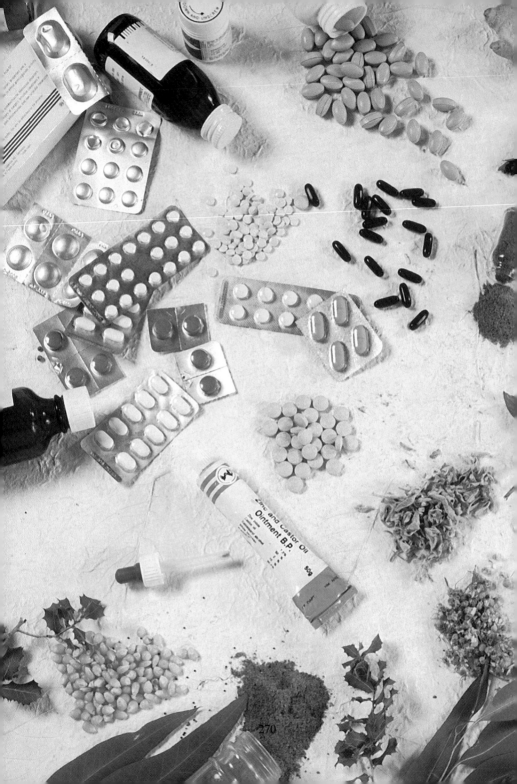

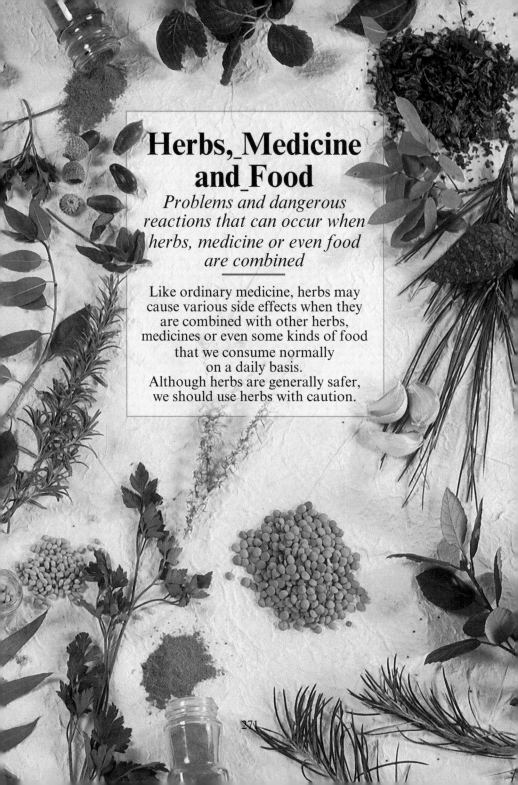

# Herbs, Medicine and_Food

*Problems and dangerous reactions that can occur when herbs, medicine or even food are combined*

Like ordinary medicine, herbs may cause various side effects when they are combined with other herbs, medicines or even some kinds of food that we consume normally on a daily basis.
Although herbs are generally safer, we should use herbs with caution.

A lot of people are under the impression that herbs are always safe to be used, since they come directly from nature. Unfortunately, this is not exactly correct. There are situations when herbs or food may interact with medications resulting to various side effects, sometimes quite serious. Even if you don't suffer from any disease, it is always wise to consult a doctor before using a herb. And you should always be alert for any unusual symptoms you did not have in the past. Even a small change in the way our body functions might be a warning of an interaction between herbs and medications.

Specialists agree today that everything natural does not necessarily mean it is safe. There is always a possibility that anything we eat may interact with another substance present in our body. The medications we use follow the same route as the foods and drinks we consume. Some medications or herbs affect the ability of the body to absorb the nourishing substances from the food we eat. Similarly, some herbs or even food we eat can decrease or increase the effectiveness of a medication.

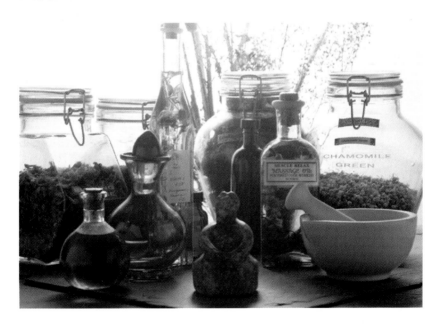

## INTERACTION - SIDE EFFECTS

We all know that alcohol interacts with almost all medications, especially with antidepressants and other medication that affect the operation of the brain or the nervous system. Some food ingredients may also increase the risk of side effects as a result of their combination with a certain medication. For example, Theophiline is a medication used for treating asthma. It contains some substances called xanthenes 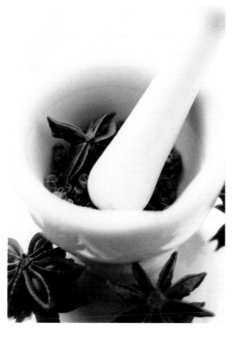 that are also present in tea, coffee, chocolate and other sources of caffeine. The consumption of large quantities of these substances in addition to Theophiline increases the risk of poisoning.

Even vitamins, food supplements and minerals may interact with other medication. Large quantities of broccoli, spinach or other green vegetables rich in vitamin K, which promote the formation of blood gloats in the arteries, reduce the effectiveness of certain medication that are used for the dilution of these blood gloats in the blood, like Heparin, Intrarfarin and others.

Some natural fibers affect the absorption of some medications. For example, fibers that are digested by the peptic system reduce the absorption of a widely spread painkiller, acetaminophen. On the other hand, fibers that are not digested by the peptic system have a similar effect on dicoxin, a medication taken by patients suffering from cardiovascular diseases.

So, since the use of herbs continues to increase, caution should be taken before combining any herbs with medications or even food. Of course there are herbs for which there are no reports of interaction or the symptoms are so mild that most of the times are not even noticed, so don't panic when you are about to use a herb. People under treatment with certain medications should be more careful.

High risk patients, like old people, patients that take three or more medications for long periods of time, diabetics, hypertensive people, patients with heart disease or high cholesterol and people suffering from depression should take extra caution and report any significant symptom or side effect to their doctor.

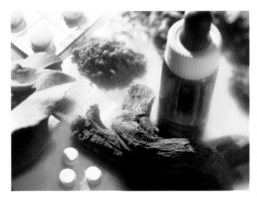

## INTERACTION OF HERBS AND DRUGS

The paragraphs that follow include some examples of the interactions of some widely used herbs with certain medications.

Hawthorn has the properties to expand the arteries and strengthen the heart muscle and is used effectively for heart diseases. It is recommended not to combine this herb with any medication containing digoxin (such as Lanoxin) which although it has similar properties, its interaction will reduce the heart beat very much, so much that it might even cause a heart attack.

According to some clinical studies, Ginseng may increase the blood pressure so it is not recommended to people trying to reduce their high blood pressure. Ginseng, Garlic and Ginger may also cause hemorrhages if they are combined with anti-coagulants like Coumadin. Coumadin is a very strong drug and people using it should always consult their doctor before taking any herb or any other drug. In some cases, Ginseng may cause over-stimulation that may result in insomnia. The combination of Ginseng and coffee or other substances that contain caffeine may again cause over-stimulation and stomach upset. In women, the prolonged use of Ginseng may cause menstrual problems and loosening of the breast.

Garlic pills or tablets may cause over-reduction of the sugar level in the blood of diabetics when combined with diabetic medication. On the other hand, there are people who are very sensitive to Garlic and its combination with certain foods may cause increased stomach acidity, gases and flatulence. Garlic has anti-coagulant properties but if it is to be combined with medications that is also anti-coagulant we should seek professional advice.

St John's Wort is a herb whose use has been rapidly increasing for the treatment of mild to moderate depression. The active ingredient in the herb is hypericin that is considered to act in a similar way upon the brain as some chemical antidepressants, known as MAO Inhibitors, do. The combination of MAO Inhibitors with foods containing the amino acid tyramine results to a very dangerous interaction. The symptoms from such an interaction vary from dizziness, sudden blood pressure increase, strong headache and sometimes fainting or even death. These symptoms appear only a few minutes after the interaction. Foods high in tyramine are old cheeses, chicken liver, various red wines, smoked meat, salted or pickled fish, beer and legumes. Therefore, since St John's Wort has similar properties to MAO Inhibitors, it is better to avoid its combination with the foods mentioned above.

There are reports, which confirm that St John's Wort has caused over-stimulation, dizziness, confusion and palpitations when it was combined with antidepressant medications. It also has the tendency to increase the blood pressure.

Willow bark is a herb that is traditionally used for fevers, headaches, rheumatic and other pains. Studies have proved that prolonged use of the

Herb may cause gastric problems and even stomach ulcers. Its side effects are similar to aspirin which was originally developed from willow bark- so the combination of the two increases their effect.

## FOOD AND MEDICATION

Medications may also interact with foods not only herbs. There are certain kinds of food that when combined with medications, they will interact with dangerous results. Patients under treatment with digoxin should avoid **Licorice** (which contains Glycyrrhizin). The combination of the two may cause heart arrhythmia and even heart attack. Also, the combination of Licorice with diuretic medications reduces the potassium levels, something that may cause weakness, numbness, muscle pains and even paralysis. Licorice also interacts with medications that reduce high blood pressure.

**Grapefruit juice** interacts with medications that control the cholesterol levels in the blood, various psychiatric drugs, contraceptives and anti-allergic drugs like Seldane, Hismanal.

**Orange juice** should not be consumed in combination with antioxidants that contain aluminium, because it increases the absorption of aluminium. The combination of orange juice and milk should also be avoided in general but especially with patients who are under treatment with antibiotic medication. The acidity of the juice reduces the effectiveness of the antibiotics and milk also has the same effect.

**Milk** should never be combined with laxatives that contain **bisacodyl** (Correctol, Dulcolax) because it increases extremely the laxative properties of the drugs.

Beverages that contain **caffeine** combined with asthma medications may cause over-excitement and palpitations.

People that are treated with **Tagament** (Simetidine) or antibiotics with **quinolone** (Cipro, Penetrex, Noroxin) or **contraceptives** should know that a cup of coffee for them equals to three.

**Grilled meat** is not recommended to Asthmatic people treated with theophylline. The chemical substances created when the meat is grilled obstruct in a way the correct function of the medication and sometimes this combination may result to unexpected asthmatic seizures.

People treated with medications for arthritis or inflammations should avoid **foods rich in fats** because this combination may affect the liver and provoke sleeplessness.

Even over the counter medications that are considered to be harmless may interact with food or other medication.

**Aspirin** for example can affect the effectiveness of steroids, diuretics and medications for arthritis. The combination of aspirin with medications for diabetes may reduce the sugar level in the blood to extremely low levels. It is very toxic when taken with drugs that fight glaucoma and epilepsy, while they may provoke hemorrhages when combined with anticoagulants such as Coumadin.

**Alcohol** interacts with the majority of medications but in cases of benzodiapezines and antidepressants it increases the drugs' effect, something that may result to unexpected conditions. Anyway, it is better not to drink alcohol in combination with drugs, any drugs. It should be also noted that foods rich in antioxidants and Beta-Carotene increase the negative effect of the alcohol on the liver.

The widely used painkillers **Acetaminophen** may cause serious damage to the liver when combined with alcohol while if they are combined with Coumadin the combination may cause internal hemorrhages.

**Antioxidants** may reduce the effectiveness of the drugs by as much as 90% when combined with antibiotics, medications that reduce high blood pressure, heart and thyroid medications.

Antibiotics and steroids reduce the effectiveness of **contraceptive**

**pills** when combined.

Various **antihistaminic drugs** like Actifed, Tarist, Theraflu, Dimetapp, Benadryl and Comtrex must be avoided by people that take tranquilisers and antidepressant medication.

**Tomatoes** and **tomato juice** contain small substances of solanine, a toxic substance that may cause headache to people that have the trend. They are also considered to be one of the most common causes of allergies. Finally, an unknown yet substance in tomatoes and their juice increases the acidity of the stomach that may result to indigestion and sourness.

**Strawberries, blackberries** and **spinach** contain oxalic acid that may irritate the liver and the cyst increasing the chances of stone formation and reduces the ability of the body to absorb sodium and iron.

The kernels of certain fruits like **apples, peaches, quinces** and **apricots** contain amygdaline, a substance that is converted into Hydrogen Cyanide in the stomach. Eating large quantities of these kernels may cause cyanide poisoning which is very dangerous.

**Potatoes** with greenish skin and small rhizomes must never be consumed. First of all they have a bitter taste, but if you don't mind the taste you should be concerned about the salonine they contain which may upset the whole organism.

Some fruits like **plums, peaches** and **apricots** are often considered to be the source of certain allergies. Clinical studies have proved that people allergic to aspirin are also allergic to those fruits, which all contain salicyline.

# DISEASE INDEX

**ABSCESSES**
Borage
Fig Tree
Flax
Nettle
Walnut

**ACME**
Cardamon
Cleavers
Flax
Soapwort
Yarrow

**AGUE**
Buckbean
Nettle

**ALLERGIES**
Balm

**ALZHEIMER**
Ginseng

**AMNESIA**
Balm
Ginseng

**ANAEMIA**
Angelica
Buckbean
Green Tea
Onion
Red Clover
Saffron
Thyme
Vine
Yellow Dock

**ANGINA PECTORIS**
Hawthorn

**ANOREXIA**
Angelica

Artichoke
Celery
Coriander
Cumin
Gentian
Ginseng
Onion
Red Clover
Wormwood

**ANTIEMETIC**
Clove
Peppermint
Quince

**ANTI-INFLAMMATORY**
Barley
Chamomile
Corn
Couchgrass
Daisy
Licorice
Willow

**ANTISEPTICS**
Eucalyptus
Lavender
Nutmeg
Olive
Oregano
Rosemary
Thyme

**ANTISPASMODICS**
Balm
Chamomile
Licorice
Valeriana
Willow

**ANXIETY**
Hawthorn
Sage

St John's Wort
Valeriana

**APHRODISIACS**
Cinnamon
Clove
Ginseng
Onion
Quince

**APPETIZERS**
Basil
Celery
Cherry
Chestnut
Chicory
Dill
Gentian
Milk Thistle
Nutmeg
Oregano
Saffron
Yellow Dock

**ARRHYTHMIA**
Hawthorn

**ARTERIOSCLEROSIS**
Garlic
Ginseng
Hawthorn
Linden
Sunflower

**ARTHRITIS**
Agrimony
Angelica
Barley
Buckbean
Celery
Chamomile
Chestnut
Clove
Elder

279

Eucalyptus
Grapefruit
Ivy
Laurel Bay
Lemon
Linden
Nettle
Oregano
Peach
Poplar
Rosemary
Soapwort
Sunflower
Thyme
Watermelon
Willow

**ASTHMA**
Anise
Cherry
Eucalyptus
Fig Tree
Garlic
Lavender
Lettuce
Licorice
Nettle
Oregano
Peach
Saffron
St John's Wort

**BACK PAINS**
Clove

**BAD BREATH**
Burning Bush
Clove
Coriander
Dill
Fennel
Nutmeg

**BAD JOINTS**
Buckbean
Chamomile

Coriander

**BEE BITES**
Agrimony

**BLEEDING**
Blackberry
Burning Bush
Cleavers
Knotgrass
Nettle
Oak Tree
Peach
Walnut

**BLOOD
CIRCULATION**
Artichoke
Cherry
Ginseng
Mustard
Nutmeg
Rosemary
Thyme
Vine

**BLOOD CLEANSERS**
Agrimony
Apple
Strawberry

**BRAIN STIMULATION**
Balm
Rosemary

**BRONCHITIS**
Anise
Borage
Cherry
Cinnamon
Ivy
Lavender
Licorice
Mallow
Marshmallow
Mustard

Nettle
Oregano
Peach
Pine
Red Clover
St John's Wort
Thyme

**BRUISES**
Agrimony
Buckbean
Daisy
Fennel
Laurel Bay
Marjoram
Mustard
Pine
Rosemary
St John's Wort

**BURNS**
Almond
Carrot
Fennel
Flax
Ivy
Lavender
Mallow
Peach
Pumpkin
St John's Wort
Strawberry

**CANCER**
Anise
Basil
Carrot
Chestnut
Garlic
Grapefruit
Green Tea
Red Clover

**CHILBLAIN**
Quince

**CHOLERA**
Clove

**CHOLESTEROL**
Artichoke
Garlic
Grapefruit
Green Tea
Olive
Sunflower

**COCITIS**
Cherry
Ivy
Oak Tree
Red Clover

**COLD**
Agrimony
Borage
Carrot
Daisy
Elder
Eucalyptus
Flax
Licorice
Mustard
Peppermint
Saffron
Sunflower
Willow
Yarrow

**COLIC**
Almond
Anise
Carrot
Chamomile
Coriander
Cumin
Dill
Fennel
Knotgrass
Lettuce
Parsley
Peppermint

St John's Wort
Walnut

**COLITIS**
Marshmallow
Rosemary

**CONFUSION**
Chrysanthemum

**CONGESTIVE HEART FAILURE**
Garlic
Hawthorn

**CONSTIPATION**
Agrimony
Apple
Arbutus
Buckbean
Chicory
Corn
Elder
Fig Tree
Flax
Linden
Mustard
Olive
Peach
Pumpkin
Quince
Strawberry

**COUGH**
Agrimony
Almond
Anise
Basil
Cherry
Elder
Eucalyptus
Fig Tree
Flax
Lemon
Lettuce
Licorice

Mallow
Marshmallow
Pine
Quince
Red Clover
St John's Wort
Sunflower

**CYST**
Apple
Carrot
Corn

**CYSTITIS**
Agrimony
Arbutus
Corn
Couchgrass
Eucalyptus
Lavender
Linden
Nettle
Peach
Pine
Yarrow

**DANDRUF**
Lemon
Rosemary
Walnut

**DEPRESSION**
Basil
Ginseng
Lavender
Pine
Rosemary
Saffron
Sage
St John's Wort
Thyme

**DIABETES**
Agrimony
Almond
Apple

Artichoke
Blackberry
Cherry
Chicory
Ginseng
Licorice
Onion
Rosemary
Sunflower
Yellow Dock

## DIARRHEA
Agrimony
Blackberry
Carrot
Chamomile
Chestnut
Cinnamon
Eucalyptus
Fig Tree
Green Tea
Knotgrass
Oak Tree
Oregano
Pomegranage
Poplar
Quince
Rose
Rosemary
Saffron
Strawberry
Vine
Walnut
Wormwood

## DIURETICS
Almond
Corn
Couchgrass
Laurel Bay
Pumpkin
Watermelon

## DIZZINESS
Balm
Lavender

Rose
Wormwood

## DROPSY
Buckbean
Carrot
Celery
Cleavers
Elder
Lettuce
Linden

## DYSENTERY
Arbutus
Basil
Blackberry
Carrot
Cinnamon
Ivy
Oak Tree
Pomegranate
Quince
Saffron
St John's Wort
Strawberry
Walnut
Yellow Dock

## DYSPEPSIA
Buckbean
Chamomile
Cherry
Cumin
Gentian
Marshmallow

## EAR INFECTIONS
Ivy
Mallow

## ECZEMA
Chamomile
Lavender
Nettle
Red Clover
Soapwort

Walnut
Yarrow
Yellow Dock

## EPILEPSY
Valeriana
Wormwood

## EXHAUSTION
Gentian
Ginseng
Onion
Sage
Strawberry
Vine

## EYE IRRITATION
Apple
Borage
Chamomile
Cherry
Chestnut
Chicory
Coriander
Elder
Fennel
Peppermint
Quince
Rose
Saffron
Watermelon

## FAINTING
Lavender
Wormwood

## FALLING HAIR
Laurel Bay
Nettle
Nettle
Olive
Rosemary
Soapwort
Walnut
Yarrow

**FAT ACCUMULATION**
Basil
Fennel
Grapefruit
Thyme

**FATIGUE**
Angelica
Cinnamon
Licorice
Rosemary
Thyme

**FEVER**
Agrimony
Almond
Apple
Arbutus
Balm
Basil
Borage
Buckbean
Chamomile
Chestnut
Chrysanthemum
Coriander
Cumin
Daisy
Elder
Eucalyptus
Laurel Bay
Lemon
Mustard
Olive
Pomegranate
Sage
Strawberry
Watermelon
Willow
Yarrow

**FIBROMYALGIA**
Ginseng

**FLATULENCE**
Anise
Arbutus
Cardamon
Carrot
Coriander
Cumin
Laurel Bay
Nutmeg
Oregano
Parsley
Peppermint
Rosemary
Saffron

**FLU**
Arbutus
Cinnamon
Eucalyptus
Lavender
Licorice
Mustard
Peppermint
Sunflower
Thyme
Willow

**FRACTURES**
Agrimony

**FRECKLES**
Cleavers
Lemon
Linden

**GALLSTONES**
Agrimony
Arbutus
Artichoke
Borage
Chicory
Cleavers
Couchgrass
Ivy
Marshmallow
Nettle
Nutmeg
Pine

Sunflower
Vine

**GASTRIC ULCER**
Barley
Licorice

**GASTRITIS**
Blackberry
Chicory
Clove
Licorice
Marshmallow
Sage
Willow

**GINGIVITIS**
Blackberry
Cardamon
Fennel
Fig Tree
Green Tea
Marshmallow
Sage

**GLAND SWELLING**
Angelica

**GONORRHOEA**
Arbutus
Poplar

**GOUT**
Buckbean
Celery
Saffron

**HEADACHE**
Balm
Burning Bush
Chrysanthemum
Coriander
Daisy
Green Tea
Lavender
Linden

Marjoram
Mustard
Quince
Rose
Rosemary
Sage
Thyme
Willow
Wormwood

**HEART**
Balm
Cherry
Cumin
Garlic
Gentian
Hawthorn
Lavender
Rosemary
Valeriana

**HEMORRHAGE**
Arbutus
Cleavers
Nettle
Sage
Vine

**HEMORRHOIDS**
Blackberry
Borage
Cardamon
Chestnut
Knotgrass
Marshmallow
Nettle
Oak Tree
Quince
Vine
Walnut
Yarrow
Yellow Dock

**HEPATITIS**
Licorice
Yellow Dock

**HERPES**
Elder
Eucalyptus
Walnut
Yarrow
Yellow Dock

**HICCOUGH**
Fennel

**HIGH
TRIGLYCERIDES**
Garlic
Green Tea
Olive

**HYPERAEMIA**
Cinnamon

**HYPERTENSION**
Balm
Blackberry
Chrysanthemum
Daisy
Garlic
Green Tea
Hawthorn
Lavender
Linden
Nettle
Olive
Onion
Parsley
Valeriana
Yarrow

**HYSTERIA**
Celery
Gentian

**INDIGESTION**
Anise
Apple
Balm
Basil
Borage

Cardamon
Cherry
Chicory
Clove
Cumin
Dill
Fennel
Grapefruit
Laurel Bay
Lemon
Linden
Mustard
Nutmeg
Rosemary
Saffron
Sage
Soapwort
Thyme
Wormwood
Yarrow
Yellow Dock

**INFANTILE CATARRH**
Anise
Fig Tree

**INFLAMMATIONS**
Agrimony
Chamomile
Chestnut
Dill
Elder
Poplar
Sage
St John's Wort
Willow

**IGMORITIS**
Laurel Bay

**INSECT BITES**
Agrimony
Balm
Basil
Cinnamon
Fennel

284

Mallow
Olive
St John's Wort

**INSECT REPELLANTS**
Basil
Elder
Walnut

**INSOMNIA**
Balm
Chamomile
Cleavers
Dill
Hawthorn
Lavender
Lettuce
Marjoram
Peach
Quince
Saffron
Sage
St John's Wort
Valeriana
Wormwood

**INTESTINAL
SWELLING**
Dill
Fennel
Mallow
Oregano
Thyme

**INTESTINE ULCER**
Chamomile
Cleavers
Fennel
Marshmallow

**ITCHING**
Peach
Soapwort

**JAUNDICE**
Carrot

Chicory
Couchgrass
Flax
Lettuce
Marshmallow
Parsley
Soapwort
Yellow Dock

**KIDNEY DISEASES**
Agrimony
Apple
Cinnamon
Elder
Linden
Parsley
Soapwort

**KIDNEY STONES**
Apple
Borage
Carrot
Corn
Dill
Lettuce
Parsley
Peach
Sunflower
Watermelon

**LARYNGITIS**
Mallow
Marshmallow
Oak Tree
Sage

**LAXATIVES**
Buckbean
Fig Tree
Flax
Licorice
Mustard
Olive
Peach
Pumpkin
Vine

**LEUCORRHOEA**
Rose
St John's Wort
Thyme

**LICE**
Anise

**LIP PARALYSIS**
Chrysanthemum

**LIVER**
Agrimony
Artichoke
Borage
Carrot
Chicory
Cinnamon
Daisy
Gentian
Grapefruit
Green Tea
Licorice
Linden
Marshmallow
Wormwood

**LIVER CIRRHOSIS**
Licorice

**LIVER
INSUFFICIENCY**
Almond
Wormwood

**LUNG DISEASES**
Basil
Borage
Eucalyptus
Nettle

**MALE IMPOTENCE**
Cinnamon
Clove
Ginseng
Onion

**MEASLES**
Cleavers
Sage

**MELANCHOLY**
Balm
Cinnamon

**MEMORY**
Anise

**MENOPAUSE**
Angelica
Saffron
Vine
Yarrow

**MENSTRUAL PROMOTION**
Carrot
Celery
Chamomile
Fennel
Oregano
Yarrow

**MENSTRUAL CRAMPS**
Balm
Chamomile
Saffron

**MENSTRUAL PAINS**
Angelica
Cinnamon
Parsley
Peppermint
Thyme
Vine

**MENTAL EXHAUSTION**
Ginseng
Onion

**MILK PRODUCTION (PROMOTE)**
Cumin
Fennel
Milk Thistle

**MIGRAINE**
Agrimony
Almond
Balm
Lavender
Linden
Thyme

**MOUTH INFECTIONS**
Cardamon
Chamomile
Fennel
Fig Tree
Marshmallow
Nettle
Rose
Sage

**MOUTH ULCERS**
Chamomile
Rose
Sage
Walnut

**MUSCLE PAINS**
Rosemary
Yarrow

**NAUSEA**
Balm
Clove
Fennel
Nutmeg
Peppermint
Pumpkin

**NEPHRITIS**
Apple

**NERVOUS BREAKDOWN**
Almond
Ginseng
Hawthorn
Lavender

**NERVOUS DISORDERS**
Burning Bush
Lavender
Valeriana

**NERVOUSNESS**
Celery
Gentian
Valeriana

**NEURALGIAS**
Chrysanthemum
Coriander
Eucalyptus
Garlic
Ivy
Laurel Bay
Mustard
Nutmeg
Rosemary
Valeriana

**NEURITIS**
Agrimony

**NOSE BLEEDING**
Knotgrass
Nettle

**ORCHITIS**
Cumin

**OSTEOARTHRITIS**
Buckbean
Willow

**OTITIS**
Ivy

286

**PAINFUL URINATION**
Knotgrass

**PALPITATIONS**
Balm
Cherry
Cumin
Parsley
Quince
Valeriana

**PHARYNGITIS**
Agrimony
Apple
Blackberry
Elder
Fig Tree
Marshmallow
Oak Tree
Sage

**PHLEBITIS**
Ivy
Vine

**PITUITARY GLANDS**
Agrimony

**PLEURISY**
Borage

**PNEUMONIA**
Borage
Elder
Flax
Mustard
Pine

**POISONING**
Basil
Fennel
Lavender
Marshmallow

**POLIO VIRUS**
Chamomile

**PROSTATE**
Almond
Anise
Arbutus
Corn
Couchgrass
Grapefruit
Onion
Pumpkin
Watermelon

**PSORIASIS**
Angelica
Cinnamon
Marshmallow
Red Clover
Yellow Dock

**QUINCY**
Sage

**RABBIES**
Gentian

**RHEUMATISM**
Agrimony
Almond
Apple
Borage
Buckbean
Celery
Chestnut
Chrysanthemum
Coriander
Corn
Elder
Eucalyptus
Fennel
Flax
Knotgrass
Laurel Bay
Lemon
Lettuce
Linden
Marjoram
Mustard

Nettle
Nutmeg
Onion
Oregano
Peach
Pine
Poplar
Soapwort
Thyme
Watermelon
Willow

**RHEUMATOID ARTHRITIS**
Buckbean
Willow

**SCABBIES**
Anise
Yellow Dock

**SCIATICA**
Rosemary

**SKIN INFECTIONS**
Burning Bush
Carrot
Chamomile
Flax
Lavender
Oak Tree
Pine
Pomegranate
St John's Wort
Thyme
Vine
Walnut
Yellow Dock

**SKIN CRACKS**
Olive
Quince
Red Clover
Soapwort

**SKIN RUSHES**
Agrimony
Almond
Blackberry
Cinnamon
Cleavers
Coriander
Fig Tree
Pumpkin

**SKIN TUMORS**
Barley
Carrot
Fig Tree
St John's Wort

**SKIN ULCERS**
Agrimony
Carrot
Sage

**SMALL POX**
Cleavers
Fig Tree
Vine

**SNAKEBITES**
Agrimony
Cinnamon
Cleavers
Fennel

**SORE THROAT**
Agrimony
Coriander
Elder
Eucalyptus
Fig Tree
Ivy
Lemon
Mustard
Pomegranate
Poplar
Quince
Sage

Yarrow
**SPLEEN**
Chicory
Gentian
Linden
Milk Thistle

**STAPHYLOCOCUS**
Onion

**STOMACH GASES**
Marjoram
Oregano
Peppermint

**STOMACH PAIN**
Agrimony
Anise
Barley
Burning Bush
Coriander
Dill
Laurel Bay
Oregano
Peach
Peppermint
Pomegranate
Poplar

**STOMACH SOURNESS**
Almond
Apple
Chamomile

**STOMACH ULCER**
Blackberry
Chamomile
Corn
Gentian
Peppermint

**STOMATITIS**
Marshmallow

**STRESS**
Ginseng
Lavender
Marjoram
Rosemary
Sage
St John's Wort
Thyme
Valeriana

**STRESS**
Chamomile
Ginseng
Lavender
Marjoram
Peppermint
Rosemary
Sage
St John's Wort
Thyme
Valeriana

**SUNBURN**
Carrot
Cleavers
Strawberry
Watermelon

**SWEATING**
Sage

**SWELLINGS**
Agrimony
Borage
Buckbean
Cinnamon
Fennel

**SYPHILIS**
Soapwort

**TAPEWORM**
Pomegranate
Pumpkin

## THORNS
Agrimony

## THROMBOSIS
Angelica
Barley
Garlic
Hawthorn
Ivy
Lemon
Onion
Yarrow

## TONIC HERBS
Arbutus
Balm
Borage
Cinnamon
Cumin
Elder
Gentian
Ginseng
Laurel Bay
Lavender
Licorice
Marjoram
Pine
Rosemary
Yellow Dock

## TOOTHACHE
Anise
Burning Bush
Clove
Daisy
Fig Tree
Ivy
Oregano

## TONSILLITIS
Agrimony
Oak Tree
Rose
Sage

## TONGUE PARALYSIS
Chrysanthemum

## TONGUE INFLAMMATIONS
Sage

## TUBERCULOSIS
Lavender
Oregano

## TYPHOID
Lemon

## URAEMIA
Knotgrass
Watermelon

## URETHRITIS
Corn
Couchgrass

## URIC ACID
Balm

## VAGINAL INFECTIONS
Chamomile
Pine

## VARICOSE VEINS
Chestnut
Ivy
Vine

## VISION
Carrot
Chrysanthemum
Daisy
Fennel
Sunflower

## VOMITING
Basil
Nutmeg

## WEIGHT LOSING
Apple
Fennel
Grapefruit
Wormwood

## WHOOPING COUGH
Almond
Fig Tree
Red Clover
Sunflower

## WOMB BLEEDING
Arbutus

## WOUNDS
Agrimony
Balm
Blackberry
Carrot
Chestnut
Cleavers
Clove
Daisy
Fennel
Ivy
Lavender
Mallow
Olive
Peach
Poplar
Pumpkin
Sage
St John's Wort
Walnut
Yarrow

## WRIGGLES
Elder
Linden

# BIBLIOGRAPHY

This book is the result of an in depth research from a group of contributors. Amongst other sources, this research included the study of various books, magazines, medical articles and announcements and the Internet. Some of the sources used are the following:

*"100 Herbs, 1000 Treatments"*, Costas Bazeos, 1998
*"Herbal Healing"*, Prineas - Sfakianakis
*"Cunningham's Encyclopaedia of Magical Herbs"*, Scott Cunningham, 1985
*"Cyclopaedia of Botanical Drugs and Preparations"*, R.C. Wren, 1982
*"Dictionary of Materia Medica"*, John H. Clarke, 1991
*"Dioscourides on Pharmacy and Medicine"*, John M. Riddle
*"Illustrated Botanical Dictionary"*, Demetrios Kavvadas, 1938
*"Field Guide to Edible Wild Plants"*, Bradford Angier, 1974
*"Handbook of Bach Flower Remedies"*, Philip M. Chancellor, 1971
*"Herbal Drugs and Phytopharmaceuticals"*, Norman Grainger Bisset, 1997
*"Medizinal - Pflanzen"*, Franz Eugen Köhler, 1887
*"Mon Herbier De Santé"*, Maurice Messegué, 1983)
*"Nature's Medicine: Plants that Heal"*, Joel L. Swerdlow, 2000
*"Nature's Prozac"*, Judith Sachs - Lendon Smith, 1998
*"Herbs, Traditional Pharmacology and Treatment"*, Anagnostopoullos, 1961
*"Vegetables"*, Mirsini Lambraki, 1997
*"The Book of Herbs"*, Hall Dorothy, 1972
*"The New Holistic Herbal"*, David Hoffman, 1991
*"Traité des Arbrisseaux et des Arbustes"*, J.H. Jaume Saint-Hilaire, 1924
*"Wild flowers of Cyprus"*, George Sfikas, 1993